Herbology in
Three Traditional
Medicines for Acne

Herbology in Three Traditional Medicines for Acne

Dr. Shuang Chen, M.D., R.H.

Library of Congress Control Number:		2011918759
ISBN:	Hardcover	978-1-4653-8274-0
	Softcover	978-1-4653-8273-3
	Ebook	978-1-4653-8275-7

This book was printed in the United States of America.

To order additional copies of this book, contact:
Xlibris Corporation
1-888-795-4274
www.Xlibris.com
Orders@Xlibris.com
103980

CONTENTS

DEDICATION

This book is dedicated to all those interested in searching for more effective single or multi-herbal formulas for use in Western, Ayurvedic, and Chinese Traditional Medicine(CTM) for the treatment of acne. It is directed to colleagues, students, patients, and all those who favor herbal medicine.

PREFACE

Acne is a common skin disorder. Some cases are effectively treated via conventional medicine, but many others are not. This book offers a reference source to provide dermatological professionals with one more option in treating patients with acne.

Herbs of Europe, North and South America, Australia, and of Chinese origin, as well as those employed in Ayurvedic Medicine, have been used locally for at least hundreds if not thousands of years to treat acne. They have enriched the experiences of herbalists in practices in many countries. Herbology is a worldwide trove of immense scientific knowledge that should be shared by all. I feel an obligation to introduce others to the extensive historical herbalistic experience in the treatment of acne. I believe that today, more and more people prefer herbal medicine for pre-illness issues and disease, and that this is becoming a growing and irreversible trend. Herbology is an important complement to the conventional treatment of acne and other disorders.

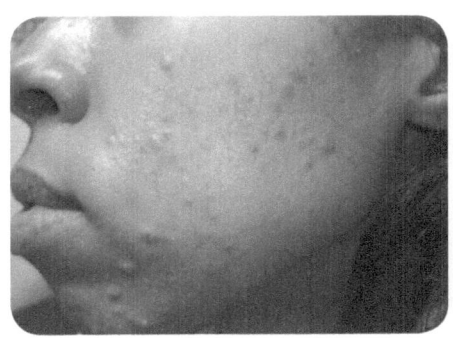
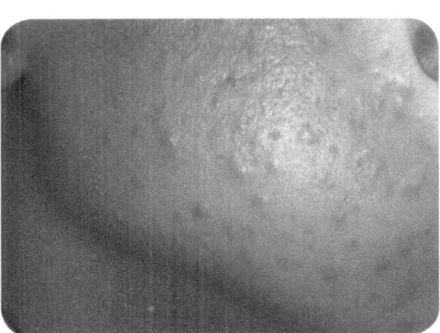

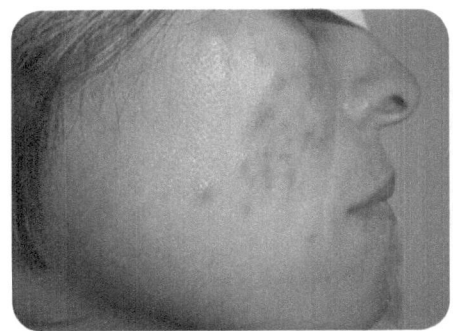
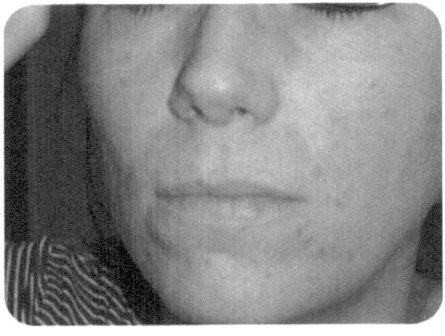

Acne

Definition

Acne is a common skin disease characterized by pimples on the face, chest, and back. It occurs when the pores of the skin become clogged with oil, dead skin cells, and bacteria.

Description

Acne vulgaris, the medical term for common acne, is the most common skin disease. It affects nearly 17 million people in the US. While acne can arise at any age, it usually begins at puberty and worsens during adolescence. Nearly 85% of people develop acne at some time between the ages of 12-25 years. Up to 20% of woman develop mild acne. It is also found in some newborns.

The sebaceous glands lie just beneath the skin's surface. They produce an oil called sebum, the skin's natural moisturizer. These glands and the hair follicles within which they are found are called sebaceous follicles. These follicles open onto the skin through pores. At puberty, increased levels of androgens (male hormones) cause the glands to produce too much sebum. When excess sebum combines with dead, sticky skin cells, a hard plug, or comedo, forms that blocks the pore. Mild noninflammatory acne consis of the two types of comedones, whiteheads and blackheads.

Moderate and severe inflammatory types of acne result after the plugged follicle is invaded by *Propionibacterium acnes*, a bacterium that normally lives on the skin. A pimple forms when the damaged follicle weakens and bursts open, releasing sebum, bacteria, and skin and white blood cells into the surrounding tissues. Inflamed pimples near the skin's surface are called papules; when deeper, they are called pustules. The most severe type of acne consists of cysts (closed sacs) and nodules (hard swellings). Scarring occurs when new skin cells are laid down to replace damaged cells.

The most common sites of acne are the face, chest, shoulder, and back since these are the parts of the body where the most sebaceous follicles are found.

Causes and Symptoms

The exact cause of acne is unknown. Several risk factors have been identified:

- Age. Due to the hormonal changes they experience, teenagers are more likely to develop acne.
- Gender. Boys have more severe acne and develop it more often than girls.
- Disease. Hormonal disorders can complicate acne in girls.
- Heredity. Individuals with a family history of acne have greater susceptibility to the disease.
- Hormonal changes. Acne can flare up before menstruation, during pregnancy, and menopause.
- Diet. No foods cause acne, but certain foods may cause flare-ups.
- Drugs. Acne can be a side effect of drugs including tranquilizers, antidepressants, antibiotics, oral contraceptives, and anabolic steroids.
- Personal hygiene. Abrasive soaps, hard scrubbing, or picking at pimples will make them worse.
- Cosmetics. Oil-based makeup and hair sprays worse acne.
- Environment. Exposure to oils and greases, polluted air, and sweating in hot weather aggravate acne.
- Stress. Emotional stress may contribute to acne.

Acne is usually not conspicuous, although inflamed lesions may cause pain, tenderness, itching, or swelling. The most troubling aspects of these lesions are the negative cosmetic effects and potential for scarring. Some people, especially teenagers, become emotionally upset about their condition, and have problems forming relationships or keeping jobs.

PHYSICAL EXAMINATION

- Lesions in areas w/ abundant sebaceous follicles: face, back, upper chest wall,
- closed comedos (whitehead) & open comedos (blackhead),

- inflammatory papules, pustules, nodules & cysts.
- Draining sinuses
- Post-inflammatory scars
- Hormonal component: flares w/menses

DIFFERENCIATIAL DIAGNOSIS

- Acne aestivalis
- Rosacea
- Steroid acne
- Perioral dermatitis
- Folliculitis
- Acne medicamentosa
- Occupational acne
- Tropical acne
- Acne cosmetic
- Syndrome of Favre-Racouchot
- Flat warts
- Trichostasis spinulosa

LABORATORY WORK-OUT

NONE

PART 1

WESTERN HERBAL MEDICINE for ACNE

A. Single Herbal Formulas for Acne

A detail introduction of **eight** single herbs for acne, some of which are approved by Commission E, some are pending approval. However all of them effectively improved or cured acne according to a number of Western herbalists' reports.

1. *Tea Tree Oil*

Scientific Name: *Melaleuca alternifolia*
Family: Myrtaceae
Common Name: Melaleuca oil, Tea tree oil

Tea tree oil is an essential oil distilled from the leaves and branches of *Melaleuca alternifolia*. A member the myrtle family (Myrtaceae), this tree is native to Australia. Australian aborigines have long used melaleuca extracts for burns, cuts, insect bites, and other skin problems. Scientists are studying melaleuca as a possible treatment for various bacterial and fungal infections. Tea tree oil contains more than 100 components, mostly monoterpene, sesquiterpenes and their alcohols. Terpien-4-ol is present at the highest level, and is responsible for most of the antimicrobial activity.

Tea tree oil was first used in surgery and dentistry in the mid-1920s. Its healing properties were also used during World War II for skin injuries to those working in munition factories. Its popularity has resurfaced with help from promotional campaigns in the past a few decades. It may be present in soaps, shampoos, lotions.

Major Compounds

Terpinenes: Primarily terpinene-4-ol (45%), gamma-terpinene(18%), alpha-terpinene (8%), 1.8-cineole (6%), alpha-terpineol (5%), as well as alpha-pinene, limonene, p-cymol, terpinolene, viridiflorene

Mechanism of Action

1. Antimicrobial Effect

    Of all of the properties claimed for tea tree oil, its antimicrobial activity has received the most attention.

    It is effective for treating acne vulgaris, and also had fewer side effects than benzoylperoxide, which showed organism *Propionibacterium acnes* was killed by terpinen-4-ol and alpha terpineol that were the major component in tea tree oil. In a separate study, tea tree oil was found to be effective against head lice.

    One study indicated that tea tree oil is similar in membrane-active disinfectants such as chlorhexidine and quaternary ammonium compounds by denaturing proteins and disrupting membrane structure. This is based on microscopic observation showing a loss of cell constituents, and breakdown of the cell wall after treatment of *E.coli* with tea tree oil as well as the observation that cells were killed prior to autolysis. Tea tree oil also able to kill *E. coli* cells in both the exponential phase and in the stationary growth. Cells in the exponential phase of growth were killed after 30 minutes of tea tree oil treatment using the known minimum bacterial concerntration of 0.25% and in the stationary phase of growth in 45 minutes using twice the minimum bacterial concentration.

    When eight components of tea tree oil were analyzed for antimicrobial activity, terpinene-4-ol inhibited all 12 of the test organisms, which were *Baccillus subtilis, Bacteriodes fragilis, Candida albicans, Clostridium perfringens, Enterococcus faecalis, Escherchia coli, Lactobacillus acidophilus, Moraxella catarrhalis, Mycobacterium smegmatis, Pseudomonas aeruginosa, Serratia marcescens,* and *Staphylococcus aureus.* Linalool and alpha-terpineol were the next most effective, killing 11 of the 12 organism. P-cymene was the least effective. The minimum cidal concentrations for linalool, terpinen-4-ol and alpha terpineol were all 0.25% or less.

Several species of Streptococcus were found to be susceptible to tea tree oil. Streptococcus pyogenes, a causative agent in impetigo, with minimum inhibitory concentration(MIC) of 0.12% tea tree oil and minimum bactericidal concentration(MBC) of 0.25%.

2. Antifungal Effect

Tea tree oil was found to be effective against Malassezia furfur, the fungal Agent implicated for pityriasis versicolor, folliculitis, and intertrigo as well as seborrheic dermatitis and dandruff. Using an agar dilution assay, 52 isolates of M. furfur gave an average MIC of tea tree oil of 0.25% after 72 hours. Using a both macrodilution assay, 16 isolates were found to have an MIC of 0.12% and a minimum antifungicidal concentration of 1.0% tea after 24 hours.

Tea tree oil was active against a variety of dermatophytes and yeast. It was able to completely inhibit the growth of Candida albicans on agar. It was diluted 1:5 in 90% ethanol and then 1:8 in agar plates. A dilution of 1:16 was MIC. It was noted that tea tree oil from different sources gave variable results.

3. Antipedicular Effect

A mixture of 50% tea tree oil and 50% of cinnamon leaf oil killed 100% of the lice and 96% the eggs. The dilution of tea tree oil alone killed 93% of the lice and 83% of the eggs.

Clinical Trials for Anti-Acne

The efficacy of a 5% topical tea tree oil gel in mild to moderate acne vulgaris was investigated in a randomized, double-blind, placebo controlled study. Sixty patients were randomly divided into two groups and treated with tea tree oil gel (n=30) or placebo (n=30) over a period of 45 days.

There was a statistically significant difference between tea tree oil and placebo in improvement of the total acne lesions count (TLC) and acne severity index (ASI).In terms of TLC and ASI tea tree oil was 3.55 times and 5.75 times more effective than placebo respectively.

A 5% solution of tea tree oil was effective in treating acne vulgaris in a study of 124 patients who were randomized to receive either tea tree oil or 5% Benzoylperoxide lotion for 3 months. It was not mentioned how often the treatment was used. Both groups showed improvement in the number of inflamed lesions, the number of noninflamed lesions, and skin oiliness.

According to more recent interviews with 62 patients recruited from Australian general practice and dermatology offices, the use of tea tree oil and other complementary and alternative therapies for acne, psoriasis, and atopic eczema is far more common than physician expected.

Clinical Trial for Toenail Fungus (Onychomycosis)

A 100% solution of tea tree oil was effective in treating onychomycosis. In this double-blind randomized trial, 117 patients with distal subungual onychomycosis, proved by culture, applied either 100% tea tree oil or 1% Clotrimazole twice daily for 6 months. At the end of 6 months, 11% of the Clotrimazole group was negative. Nail appearance improved in 61% of Clotrimazole patients and 60% of tea tree oil patients. A 3-month follow-up showed that a positive resolution was still present in 55% of the Clotrimazole patients and 56% of the tea tree oil patients.

Clinical Trial for Skin Inflammation (Histamine-induced)

Tea tree oil significantly decreased histamine-induced skin inflammation in 21 subjects 20 minutes after histamine injection in an open trial. Twenty- seven subjects were injected intradermally with histamine diphosphate (5mcg/50 mcL) on each forearm. Flare area and weal volume was calculated after measuring weal diameters and double skin thickness every 10 minutes for 1 hour. Twenty-one subjects had 25 mcL of 100% tea tree oil topically applied to one forearm at 20 minutes while 6 subjects had 25 mcL paraffin oil topically applied to a forearm. The percentage weal volume of tea tree oil treated arms was statically significantly lower than that of the control arms (p=0.0004, Mann-Whitney U-test) at 30 minutes, and at 60 minutes. (p=0.017).

Indications

Unproven uses:

> Topically for **Acne,** athlete's foot, bacterial and fungal infections of the skin, nails and mouth tissues, boils, eczema, lice, psoriasis, vaginal infections, wounds, ulcers of the oral mucus membrane, gingivitis, root canal treatment, insect bites and burns.

> Orally for Tonsillitis, pharyngitis, colitis and sinusitis.

Precautions and Adverse Reactions

- Allergic contact dermatitis
- Diarrhea
- Vomiting
- Skin irritation (in sensitive people)
- Central nervous system depression, such as excessive drowsiness, sleepiness, and inability to coordinate muscles
- Irritating mouth and digestive tract

Drug Interactions

> No human interaction data available

Warnings

- **Avoid** taking tea tree oil internally
- **Watch** the percentage of tea tree oil concentration on the label carefully, and avoid using 100% pure oil for certain skin rashes excepting the nail fungus condition.
- **Keep** tea tree oil **away** from children.
- Pregnant and breast—feeding woman **don't use** tea tree oil.
- **Avoid** tea tree oil if the person has experienced an allergy to any of its components.

Dosage

> Tea tree oil comes as creams, ointment, lotions, and soaps. It is also found in cosmetics, toiletries, and other household products. Concentration of tea tree oil in these products range from 1% to 100%.

- For acne using 5-10% tea tree oil once a day for up to one month.
- For athlete's foot, using 10% tea tree oil twice a day up to one month.
- For treating fungal infection of fingernails or toenails using 100% pure tea tree oil twice a day for at least 6 months.
- For oral candidiasis using one tablespoonful of 5% tea tree oil solution as a mouth wash taken up to 4 times a day. (make sure to spit out)

Storage

Store tightly sealed and protected from light

2. *Aloe vera*

Scientific Names: *Aloe capensis, Aloe barbadensis, and Aloe vera ferox.*
Family : Aloaceae
Common Name: Aloe

Aloe is a plant that looks like a cactus, but is actually a member of the Liliaceae family. It grows in Africa, Asia and the warmer parts of America and Europe. Aloe leaves contain a gel that is rich in therapeutic properties, which are contribute to the most important complex carbohydrate or polysaccharides called **Acemannan** and its full name is poly B-1,4 mono-acetyl mannose 1, a prominent glucomannan. This polysaccharide is found in the parenchyma of the aloe leaf, in a gelatinous structure that when separated from the aloe leave rind. Another glycoprotein with antiallergic properties, called alprogen and novel anti-inflammatory compound, C-glucosyl chromone had been isolated from aloe vera gel.

Previous studies showed that two major bio-activities of aloe are that, anti-inflammatory activity found primarily in the lower molecular weight fraction, and immunomodulatory activity found in the high molecular weight fraction.

Major components

Vitamins: vitamin A, C, E, B12, folic acid, choline;

Enzymes: brdykinase, aliiase, alkaline phosphatase, amylase, carboxypeptidase, catalase, cellulose,lipase, and peroxidase;

Minerals: calcium, copper, selenium, magnesium, manganese, potassium, sodium, zinc;

Sugars: monosaccharides (glucose/fructose) and polysaccarides(glucomannans/ polymannose);

Anthraquinones: 12 anthraquinones that includes aloin and emodin act as analgesics, antibacterials and antivirals;

Fatty acids: 4 plant steroids: cholesterol, campeterol, B-sisosterol and lupeol. They have anti-inflammatory action and lupeol also possesses antiseptic and analgestic properties;

Hormones: Auxins and gibberellins that help in wound healing and have anti-inflammatory action;

Others: It provides 20 of 22 human required amino acids and 7 of 8 essential amino acids. It also contains salicylic acid that possesses anti-inflammatory and antibacterial properties.

Mechanism of Action

Feature of healing: Glucomannon and gibberellin work together which increases collagen synthesis after topical and oral aloe vera. It not only increased collagen content of the wound but also changed collagen composition (more type III) and increased the degree of collagen cross linking. Due to this, it accelerated wound contraction and increased the breaking strength of resulting scar tissue.

Feature of anti-inflammation: It inhibits the cycloxygenase pathway and reduces prostaglandin E2 production from arachidomic acid. And the novel anti-inflammatory compound C-glucosyl chromone was isolated from aloe gel extracts.

Feature of anti-UV light damage: Aloe gel has a protective effect against radiation damage to the skin. After topical and oral aloe gel, an antioxidant protein metallothionein that is generated in the skin, which scavenges hydroxyl radicals and prevents suppression of superoxide dismutase and glutathione peroxidase in the skin. It reduces the production and release of skin keratinocyte-derived immunosuppressive cytokines such as interleukin-10 and hence prevents UV-induced suppression of delayed type hypersensitivity.

Action on the immune system: Alprogen inhibit calcium influx into mast cells, thereby inhibiting the antigen-antibody—mediated release of histamine and leukotriene from mast cells. A few low-molecular-weight compounds are capable of inhibiting the release of reactive oxygen free radicals from activated human neutrophils.

Moisturizing and anti-aging effects: Aloe stimulates fibroblast which produces the collagen and elastin fibers making the skin more elastic and less wrinkled, which due to mucopolysaccharides help in binding moisture into the skin. It also has cohesive effects on the superficial flaking epidermal sells by sticking them together, which softens the skin. The amino acids also soften the hardened skin cells and zinc acts an astringent to tighten pores.

Laxative effects: Anthraquinones present in latex are a potent laxative.

Antiviral and antitumor activity: These actions may be due to indirect or direct effects. Indirect effect is due to stimulation of the immune system and direct effect is due to anthraquinones.

Antiseptic effect: Ale vera contains 6 antiseptic agents: lupeol, salicylic acid, urea nitrogen, cinnamonic acid, phenols and sulphur. They all have inhibitory action on fungi, bacteria and viruses.

Indications:

Unproven uses: **Acne vulgaris,** skin minor burns, sun burn, abrasions, cuts, irritations, wounds, frostbite, stomach ulcers, radiation dermatitis, constipation, genital herpes, hemorrhoids, mucositis, colitis, AIDS, asthma, bleeding, arthritis, common cold, seizures, varicose veins, bursitis, depression.

Precautions and Adverse Reactions

Topical: It may cause skin irritation, redness, burning, stinging sensation and rarely generalized dermatitis in sensitive individuals. Allergic reactions are mostly due to anthraquinones, such as aloin and barbaloin. It is best to apply it to a small area first to test for possible allergic reaction. It may cause delayed healing of deep wounds also.

Oral: Abdominal cramps, red urine, hepatitis, dependency or worsening of constipation, dehydration, severe diarrhea, kidney damage even possible death, which mostly caused by overdose or large dose. Laxative effect may cause electrolyte imbalances that such as low potassium level may resulting in irregular heart beats, weakness, and flaccid muscles. If take it during late stage pregnancy, may have a risk of spontaneous abortion or premature. Also, it might cause blood build-up in the pelvis if you use large doses.

Drug Interactions

Do not use aloe internally if you are taking:

- digoxin (Lanoxin)
- drugs that cause potassium loss, such as Bunex, Demadex, Edecrin, Lasix, and Sodium Edecrin
- diuretics
- drugs for irregular heartbeats
- steroids

Warnings

Do not use external aloe preparations if patient is allergic to aloe or plants in the Lyliaceae family (such as garlic, onion, and tulips).

Do not take aloe internally if patient is pregnant, breast-feeding, or menstruating.

Do not give aloe to children.

Avoid take aloe internally if patient suffers from kidney disease or heart disease.

Avoid aloe if patient experiences severe stomach discomfort and serious problems from body salt imbalances.

Do not recommend to injecting aloe due to it reported that four people have died after receiving aloe injections for cancer.

Dosage

Oral :
Softgels: Aloe vera Extract (200:1 Concentrate), 75 mg/3 softgels equivalent to 1 tablespoon of pure aloe vera gel (15,000mg)
Dose: 3 softgels, one to three times/day
Capsules: 470mg, 1-2 caps, two to three times/day

Gel: 90%, 98%,99.5%,99.6% 2-4 oz/day
Juice: 99.6%, 99.7% 2-4 oz/day

Topical :
Cream, hair conditioner, jelly, juice, liniment, lotion, ointment, shampoo, skin cream, soap, sunscreen.

For skin irritation, itching, burns, cuts, and other wounds, apply an external form of aloe liberally as needed.

Smallest dose needed to maintain a soft stool should be used.

3. *Bittersweet nightshade*

Scientific Name: *Solanum dulcamara L.*
Family : Solanaceae (nightshades)
Common Names: Bittersweet nightshade, dulcamara, deadly nightshade, bittersweet, felonwort, violet-bloom, woody nightshade, fellen, snake berry, scarlet berry, fever twig, blue nightshade, staff vine, fellonwood, and woody.

The stem of bittersweet nightshade is good for medical use. This plant is common in Europe, northern Africa, eastern and western Asia, and North America.

Compounds:

Steroid alkaloid glycosides: (0.07-0.4%) the alkaloid spectrum varies widely with variety

Tomatidenol: variety-alpha-solamarine, beta-solamarine

Soladulcidine: variety-soladulcidinetetraoside

Solasodine: variety-solasonine, solamargine

Steroid saponins

Mixed varieties also occur.

Mechanism of Action

The main active principles are the steroid alkaloid glycoside whose resorption is probably promoted by the saponins. They stimulate phagocytosis, are hemolytic, cytotoxic, antiviral, anticholinergic, and have local anesthetic properties.

Solasodine has a cortisonelike effect. A desensitizing and cardiotonic effect has been observed in clinical trials with patients suffering from rheumatic polyarthritis.

Its use as an expectorant may be due to the saponin content.

Indications

Approved by Commission E*:

- Eczema
- Furuncles
- **Acne**
- Warts

*The German Commission E monographs.

Unproven Uses: In folk medicine, bittersweet nightshade is used internally for nose bleeds, rheumatic conditions, asthma, and bronchitis, and to stimulate the immune system; externally for herpes, eczema, abscesses, and contusions.

Homeopathic Uses: Solanum dulcamara is used for inflammation of the respiratory and gastrointestinal tracts, the joints and skin, and for febrile infections. Efficacy has not been proved.

Contraindications

Bittersweet nightshade is contraindicated in pregnancy and nursing mothers.

Precautions and Adverse Reactions

Health risks or side effects following the proper administration of designated therapeutic dosages are not recorded.

Toxic effects should not be seen in dosage under approximately 25 gram due to the low alkaloid content of the stem.

Drug Interactions

No interaction data is available.

Overdosage

The unripe berries have caused poisonings among children. More than 10 berries cause nausea, vomiting, dilated pupils, and diarrhea. Lethal dosage is estimated to be 200 berries.

Dosage

Mode of administration: Comminuted herb is used in teas and other galenic preparation for internal use. This herb is also used externally in compresses and rinses.

Preparation: A decoction is prepares by adding 1-2 gram of herbal medicine to 250 ml water.

Daily dosage:
The average daily internal dose is 1-3 gram of the herbal medicine. Externally, the herb is used as infusions or decoctions that have strengths equivalent to 1-2 gram of herbal medicine per 250 ml water.

Homeopathic Uses:
5 drops, 1 tablet, or 10 globules every 30-60 minutes (acute) or 1-3 times a day(chronic); parenterally:1-2 ml, sc, acute: 3 times daily; chronic: once a day.

4. *Heartsease*

Scientific Name: *Viola tricolor*
Family : Violaceae
Common Names: Heartsease, European wild pansy, pansy, garden violet, biddy's eyes, cat's face, field pansy, and johnny-jump-up, pansy viscum.

Heartsease is found in abundance on hedgebanks and waste ground, but it also seems to be a "weed of cultivation" that can be found freely in cornfields and garden ground. This plant is indigenous to temperature Eurasia, from the Mediterranean to India and as far as Ireland. It is cultivated in Holland and France.

It is odorless and the taste slimysweetish.

Medical Parts: The medicinal parts are the dried aerial parts, the fresh aerial parts of the flowering plant, and the whole plant.

Compounds

Flavonoinds (0.2-0.4%): including among others rutin (violaquercitrin, 23%), Luteolin-7-0-glucosides, scoparin, saponarine, violanthin, vicinein-2, vitexin.

Phenol carboxylic acid: salicylic acid(0.06-0.3%), violutoside (violutin, gluconarabinoside, of the methyl salicylate)

Mucilage(10%)

Tannins(2-5%)

Hydroxycoumarins: umbelliferone

Triterpene saponins (speculated)

Mechanism of Action

This herb medicine has soothing, salvelike effects due to its mucin content. In animal experiments, oral use brought about an improvement of eczemalike skin conditions after long-term use. The antisporiatic effect attributed to this herb may be explained by the saponin content, as can its use for catarrh of the upper respiratory tract. In vitro it is hemolytic and increases chloride elimination in the urine.

Indications
Approved by Commission E:

• Inflammation of the skin

Unproven Uses: External uses include mild seborrheic skin diseases, cradle cap in children, and various skin disorders, including wet and dry exanthema, eczema, crusta lacteal, **acne**, impetigo, and pruritus vulvae. The plant is used orally as a mild laxative for constipation and as an auxiliary agent to promote metabolism.

Homeopathic Uses: This herb is used for eczema and inflammation of the urinary tract.

Precautions and Adverse Reactions

No health hazard or side effects are known in conjunction with the proper administration of the designated therapeutic dosages.

Pregnant and lactating woman better do not use this herb orally due to it is a mild laxative.

Drug Interactions

No interaction data is available.

Dosage

Mode of Administration: Whole, cut and powdered herb is available for infusions, decoctions, and other galentic preparations. It is also available in ointments and shampoo for external use.

Preparation: To make a tea, pour 1 cup of scalding water over 1 dessertspoonful of herb. An infusion for internal use is prepared using 5-10 g herb per 1 litter of water. A decoction for internal use is prepared by adding 1.5 g herb to 1 cup water. The herb is also used as a bath additive.

Daily Dosage: A cup of tea should be taken 3 times daily after meals. The dose for the infusion is 1 dessertspoonful 3 times daily. The dose for the powdered herb is 1/2 teaspoonful in hot sugar water 3 times daily.

Homeopathic Dosage: 5 drops, 1 tablet, or 10 globules every 30-60 minutes (acute) or 1-3 times daily (chronic); parenterally: 1-2 ml sc, acute: 3 times daily; chronic: once a day.

5. German chamomile

Scientific Name: *Matricaria recutita*
Family : Asteraceae
Common Name: Chamomila, Chamomile, Hungurian chamomile, Pin heads, Single chamomile.

This herb is indigenous to Europe and northwest Asia, neutralized in North America and elsewhere.

Medical parts: The medicinal parts consist of the entire flowering herb or only the flowers.

Characteristic: The receptacle of the compound head of German Chamomile is hollow which distinguishes it from other types of Chamomile.

Habitat: German Chamomile is indigenous to Europe and northwest Asia, naturalized in North America and elsewhere.

Compounds

Volatile oil(0.4-1.5%):chiefcompounds(-)-alpha-bisabolol(levomenol),bisabolol oxide A, bisabolol oxide B, bisabololone oxide A, beta-trans-farnesene, trans-en-yne-dicycloether(polyyne spiroether, adjoining cis-en-yn-dicycloether), chamazu- lene(blue in color, arising from the non-volatile proazulene matricin after steam distillation), spathulenol

Flavonoids: flavone glycosides, aglycones apigenin, luteolin, chrysoeriol, chief Glycosides apigenin-7-O-glucoside, apigenin glucoside acetate,-flavonol glycosides, Aglycones including quercetin, isorhamnetin, patuletin, for example rutin, hyperoside.

Unbound, Highly Methoxylized Flavonoids: jaceidinem chrysospenol, chrysosplenetin

Hydroxycoumarins: including umbelliferone, herniarin

Mucilages: (10% in the mucilage ribs, fructans) including rhamanogalacturonane

Therapeutic Actions

It has shown wound-healing, antidiarrheal, sedative, anti-inflammation, anti-bacterial, anti viral, anti fungal infective properties. It shown that possesses antioxidant, antineoplastic and anxiolytic effects. It is beneficial to the skin and the gastrointestinal tract also.

Indications

Approved by Commission E*:

- Cough/ Bronchitis
- Fevers and colds
- Inflammation of the skin
- Inflammation of the mouth and pharynx
- Tendency to infection
- Wounds and burns

*The German Commission E monographs

Unproved: topically used for **acne**, furuncles, hemorrhoids, abscesses and early stage of skin infected diseases.

Precautions

- High doses of chamomile may cause allergic conjunctivitis, contact dermatitis, and eczema.
- Severe allergic reaction: chest tightness, wheezing, hives, itching, and rashes.
- Vomiting

Drug Interactions

Moderate risk:

- *Anticoagulants*: combining herbs with certain drugs may alter their action or produce unwanted side effects, especially blood thinners such as Coumadin(do not take chamomile when taking these drugs), which may result in increased risk of bleeding.
  Clinical Management: Caution is advised if used concomitantly. **Monitor** the patient for signs and symptoms of excessive bleeding.

- *Alcohol/Benzodiazepines*: may cause additive effects of alcohol and benzodiazepines.
  Clinical Management: **avoid** concomitant use.

Dosage

Mode of Administration: Liquid and solid preparations are available for external and internal application.

Orally:
Capsule: 125mg,345mg, 350mg, 354mg, 360mg
Liquid: 1:4
Oil: 100%
Tea:
Preparation: An infusion for internal use is prepared by pouring boiling water(150ml) over 3 grams of chamomile, cover for 5 to 10 minutes and strain. (1 teaspoonful = 1 gram drug).

Topically:

An infusion for topically poultice application is prepared by pouring
1½ cups of hot water over 2 dessertspoons of the drug, cover, leave to steep for 15 minutes and then strain.
Ointments and gels are available in strengths of 3 to 10%.

Daily Dosage:

An internally single dosage is approximately 3 g as an infusion. Liquid extract 1 to 4 ml or 1 cup of freshly made tea is administered 3 to 4 times daily.

Externally as a bath additive, 50g is added to 1 Litter of water or 6 g of drug for a steam bath.

Washes and gargles may be administered several times a day.

6. *Burdock*

Scientific Name: *Arctium lappa*
Family : Asteraceae (formerly Compositae)
Common Names: Burdock root, lappa, beggar's buttons, clot bur, and thorny burr, bardada, burr seed, cockle buttons, fox's clote, hardock, hareburr.

Burdock is a biennial herb and is found growing wild through North America, New Zealand, and Australia. In North America, it can be found everywhere, especially near farmyards, in vacant city lots, and along rivers. Burdock loves nitrogen rich, undisturbed soil.

Compounds

Volatile oil (small amounts) of very complex make-up: including phenylacetaldehyde, benzaldehyde, 2-alkyl-3-methoxy-pyrazines.

Lignans: neoarchtiin A

Sesquiterpene lactones

Polyynes : chief components are trideca-1, 11-dien-3,5,7,9-tetrain, as well as sulphur derivatives.

Caffeic acid derivatives: including chlorogenic acid, isochlorogenic acid.

Polysaccharides: insulin (fructose), mucilage's (xyloglucans, acidic xylans).

Triterpenes: including alpha-amyrin, omega-taraxarsterol, present to some extent as acetic acid ester.

Phytosterols: beta-sitosterol, stigmasterol, campestrol and their esters.

Tannins

Therapeutic Action

Alterative, antibiotic, anti-inflammatory, antineoplastic, antiscorbutic, antirheumatic, antiseptic, antiviral, aperient, demulcent, depurative, diaphoretic, diuretic, orexigenic, stomachic, tonic, and vulnerary.

Indications

Unproven uses:
Acne, boils, carbuncles, skin infections, cancer, canker sores, psoriasis, eczema, erythema of the skin, ichthyosis (externally apply), seborrhea of the scalp (externally apply), gout, hemorrhoids, HIV, kidney stones, cystitis, lower back pain, impotence, rheumatism, sciatica, ulcers, and blood purifying.

Chinese Medicine: Burdock is used to treat carbuncles, ulcers, and erythema of the skin as well as sore throat. Efficacy has not been proved.

Precautions

No health hazards or side effects are known in conjunction with the proper administration of designated therapeutic dosages. Giving the lack of toxicity data and reports of in-vitro uterine stimulant action, use it during pregnancy and lactation should be avoided.

Burdock can be safely combined with pharmaceutical drugs other than the combination of the any burdock tincture or alcohol extract with disulfiram or metronidazole due to the alcohol content.

Drug Interactions

No interaction data is available.

Dosage

Mode of Administration: administered as a drug and, for external use, in the form of burdock oil (extract with fat oil).

Preparation:
Tea: steep 2.5 g (1 teaspoon) of the drug with 150 ml boiling water.

Capsules: 460 mg and 475 mg
Fluid Extract: 1:1
Daily Dose: Tea: 1 cup, 1 to 2 times a day.

7. *Yellow dock*

Scientific Name: *Rumex crispus*
Family : Polygonaceae
Common Name: Curled dock, Garden patience, Sour dock, and Narrow dock

Yellow dock is a perennial flowering herb that is indigenous to Europe and Africa, but grows wild in many regions of the world.

Compounds

Oxalate: oxalic acid, calcium oxalate

Tannins (3-6%)

Flavonoids: including among others, quercitrin

Anthracene derivatives (0.9-2.5%): anthranoids, aglycones physcion, chryosphanol, Emodin, aloe-emodin, rhein, their glucosides

Naphthalene derivatives: neopodin 8-glucoside, lapodin

Therapeutic Action

Alterative, blood tonic, laxative, diuretic, cholagogue, anti-inflammatory, antibiotic.

Indications

Unproven uses:
Scabies, **acne** and other skin diseases, chronic liver congestion, constipation, fluid retention, intermitted fever, sore throat, stomach upset, swollen glands, syphilis, tonsillitis, allergy symptoms.

Precautions and Adverse Reactions

- Abdominal pain
- Nausea
- Diarrhea
- Vomiting

The mucus membrane irritation accompanied by vomiting is possible following intake of the fresh rhizome, due to its anthrones content. The anthrones are oxidized to anthraquinones after dehydration and storage. And consuming excessive amounts of this herb can cause metabolic acidosis and a severe calcium deficiency in the blood, resulting in death.

Interactions

Combining herbs with certain drugs may alter their action or produce unwanted side effects.

Warnings

Don't use it when patient is pregnant because it may cause miscarriage.

Don't use it if patient has kidney dysfunction or kidney failure, diabetes, liver disease, or a severe body salt (electrolyte) abnormality.

Use it cautiously if patient has heart failure, newly diagnosed diabetes, malnutrition, or a disease relate to alcoholism or if patient has had recent thyroid or parathyroid surgery. Also use it with caution if patient is taking drugs that decrease blood calcium, such as diuretic, Dilantin, Miacalcin, or Mithracin.

Watch for symptoms of low blood calcium, including fatigue, seizures, confusion, muscle spasm, and numbness or tingling around the mouth.

If patient is taking this herb, he or she should get blood calcium test periodically.

Don't use it instead of prescribed antiviral drugs to treat herpes or HIV.

Be aware that boiling the root too long reduces yellow dock's chemical activity.

Dosage

Capsules: 470mg, 500mg
Liquid: 1: 1

8. *Oregon grape*

Scientific Name: *Mahonia aquifolium*
Family: Berberidaceae
Common Name: Oregon grape, Holly-leaved barberry, Mountain grape

Oregon grape comes from the bark of the roots and stems of Mahonia aquifolium, a bushy shrub that grows in the thickets and pastures in the western United States. This herb gets its name from its use as a food and medicine along the Oregon trial. The shrub's fruits are used in wines and brandies.

Active Components

Oregon grape root has alkaloid that includes berberine, berbamine, canadine, hydrastine and tannins. It contains other constituents except alkaloids. Isolated berberine has been shown to effectively treat diarrhea in patients infected with E. coli, and it inhibits the ability of bacteria to attach to human cells, which helps prevent infections, particularly in the throat, intestines, and urinary tract.

In one clinical trial, an ointment of Oregon grape was found to be mildly effective for reducing skin irritation and itching in patients with mild to moderate psoriasis.

Whole Oregon gape extract were shown in one pharmacological study to reduce inflammation (Psoriasis) and stimulate the white blood cells known as macrophages. In this study, isolated alkaloids from Oregon grape didn't show these actions which indicates that certain active constituents exist besides alkaloids are to the properties of Oregon grape responsible for relieving inflammation.

Therapeutic Actions

Oregon grape has synergistic antibacterial, anti-inflammatory, and bile-stimulating properties which make the crude extract useful in acne. It has potential antimutagenic/anticarcinogenic/anticancer activity. It is hepatic, astringent, antioxidant, emetic, diuretic, cholagogue, laxative, blood purifying and relaxant also.

Indications

Unproven uses:
Acne, arthritis, as an expectorant, blood stream infection, bronchitis, diarrhea, eczema, fever, fluid retention, gallbladder disease, hepatitis, herpes, kidney stones, urinating tract infection, psoriasis, rheumatism, stomach upset, syphilis, to stimulate bile production, vaginitis.

Drug Interactions and Precautions

It interacts with certain antibiotics, such as doxycycline or tetracycline. It is not recommended with doxycycline or tetracycline for diarrhea because this herb may interfere with the intestinal ability to absorb them.

Studies show that it has berberine, which create uterine contractions and to increase levels of bilirubin. Also infere with normal bilirubin metabolism in infants, and it might worsen jaundice.

Dosage

Common doses:

- Capsules: 400 mg, 2-3 capsules per day with water at a morning or mid-day

- Tincture: each serving contains Oregon grape root fluid extract (1:1) 1000mg in 12-15% certified alcohol, ½-1.0ml 3 times per day.
- Decoction: boiling 5-15 gram of chopped roots of this herb in 2 cups of water (500ml) for 15 minutes. After straining and cooling, 3 cups (750ml) can be used per day.
- Topically: 10% Oregon grape root extract ointment/cream are applied, three times per day to the infected area.

Warnings

- Oral use of this herb not recommended to pregnant and breast-feeding women
- Do not use it if the patient has experienced an allergy to it or related herb
- Avoid getting this herb in your eyes. If do, flush your eyes with water
- Be aware that skin contact this herb may cause intense pain
- Don't confuse this herb with the common Barberry, *Berberis vulgaris*.
- Not recommended for orally use longer than 3-4 weeks.

9. *Other Single Herbs for Acne, Oral or/and Topical*

Angelica, *Angelica archangelica* (AM)
Angrimony, *Agrimonia eupatonia* (AM)
Anise, *Pimpinella anisum* (AM, IM)
Barberries, *Berberis vulgaris* root, bark, stem and flower (IM, AM)
Basil oil, *Ocimum basiliccum* oil (AM), topically only
Calendula, *Calendula officinalis,* deep orange flowered variety (IM, AM), topically
Chaparral, *Larrea tridentate, Larrea divaricata* (AM), topically
Chickweed, *Stellaria media* leaf, stem, and flower (IM, AM), topically
Cowslip, *Primula veris* (AM)
Dandelion, *Taraxacum officinale* leaf and root (AM)
Echinacea, *Echinacea angustifolia* or *E. pallid* root and rhizomes (AM,IM)
Eucalyptus, *E. golobulus and E. viminulis* oil (AM), topically only
Garlic, *Allium sativum* cloves or powder (AM)
Gentian, *Gentiana lutea* root (AM)
Goldenseal, *Hydrastis Canadensis* root (AM,IM)
Goldthread, *Coptis chinensis* root (IM, AM)
Horsetail, *Equisetum arvense* (AM)
Lemon grass, *Cymbopogon citrates* (AM)
Magnolia, *Magnolia spp.* Stem bark (IM)
Marshmallow, *Althaea officinalis* (AM,IM)
Myrrh, *Commiphora molmol* and other *Commiphora species* (AM, IM)

Neem oil, *Azadirachta indica* oil (AM), topically only
Oregon grape, *Mahonia aquifolium* root (IM,AM,AC)
Prickly ash, the Northern prickly ash *Zanthoxylum americanum* bark, and the
Southern prickly ash *Z. clava-herculis* tree (IM)
Red clover, *Trifolium pretense* rose colored flower head (AM,IM)
Sarsaparilla, *Smilax species* (*S. aristochiifolia, S.regelli, S. febrifuga, S. ornata* root) (IM)
Sassafras, Sassafras albidum root and bark (IM)
Scute, (Asian skullcap) *Scutellaria baicalensis* root (IM,AC)
Stillingia, *Stillingia sylvatica L., Euphorbiaceae* root (AM, IM)
White oak, *Quercus alba* bark (IM, AM)
Wild oregano, *Origanum vulgare* (AM, IM)
Witch hazel, *Hamamelis virginiana* leaves and bark (IM),topically only
Worm wood, *Artemista absinthium* leaf (AM)
Yarrow, *Achillea millefolium* flowering top (AM)
Yellowroot, *Xanthorrhiza simplicissima* root (IM, AM)
AC: Anti-Comedogenic herb

AM: Antimicrobial herb
IM: Inflammation-Modulating herb

B. Multi-Herb Formulas for Acne

1. Herbal formula for acne, orally and topically from ACHS*

> 1 oz/30 gm Burdock root, *Artium lappa*
> 1oz /30 gm Yellow dock root, *Rumex crispus*
> 1oz /30 gm Yarrow flowers, *Achillea millefolium*
> 1oz /30gm Marshmallow root
> 5 pints/3 liters of water

> Simmer the herbs in the water until the mixture reduces down to 3 pints/1.8 liters. Take 1 tablespoon three times a day between meals. This preparation can also be applied topically.

> *ACHS: American College of Healthcare Sciences, Portland, Oregon of USA

2. Dr. Yarnell's herbal formula for acne, orally

Oregon grape, *Mahonia aquifolium* fresh root tincture, 20-30% (IM, AM, AC);
Scute, *Scutellaria baicalensis* decocted dried root tincture, 20-30% (IM, AC);

Yarrow, *Acchillea millefolium* fresh flowering top tincture, 10-20% (IM, AM);
Turmeric, *Curcuma longa* fresh root tincture, 10-20% (IM);
Gugul, *Commiphora mukul* resin tincture, 5-10% (AC? IM?);
Licorice, *Glycyrrhiza glabra* dried root fluid extract, 5-10% (IM, AM, Flavor enhancer;
Devil's club, *Oplopanax horridum* fresh root bark glycerite, 5-10% (for stress);
Chase tree, *Vitex agnus-castus* mature fruit tincture 10-20% (hormone balancing);
Saw palmetto, *Serenoa repens* mature fruit tincture, 10-20% (if androgens are excessive).

Dose: Orally, 1 tsp three times per day in water sipped before meals

3. Dr.Christopher's herb formulas for acne, orally

Below two formulas are from Dr. John R. Christopher who was a Naturopathic Doctor and herbalist in the US.

a). Herbal formula for hormonal changing
Black cohosh, *Cimicifuga racemosa*
Licorice, *Glycyrrhiza glabra*
Sarsaparilla, *Smilax species*
False unicorn, *Chamaelirium luteum*
American ginseng, *Panax quinquefolius*
Blessed thistle, *Cnicus benedictus, Carbenia benedicta, Carduus benedictus*
Squawvine, *Mitchella repens*

Dose: 2 capsules three times a day before food.

b). Herbal formula for lower bowel cleanse
Cascara sagrada bark, *Rhamnus purshiana*
Goldenseal root, *Hydrastis canadensis*
Turkey rhubarb root, *Rheum palmatum*
Red raspberry leaf, *Rubus idaeus*
Fennel seed, *Foeniculum vulgare*
Barberry bark, *Berberis vulgaris*
Ginger root, *Zingiber officinale*
Lobelia, *Lobelia inflata*
Cayenne, *Capsicum species*, 40 MHU

Dose: 2 capsules, twice a day before food.
Above two formulas should be orally taken together.

4. Herbal Formula for Acne, oral and topical use from David Hoffmann*

Blue flag, *Iris versicolor*	1 part
Greater burdock, *Arctium lappa*	1 part
Echinacea, *Echinacea spp.*	1 part
Cleavers, *Galium aparine*	1 part

Dose: up to 5 ml of tincture three times a day. The patient should drink an infusion of stinging nettle*(Urtica dioica)* two or three times a day. In addition, apply calendula (*Calendula cofficins)* topically as a wash, in the form of an infusion mixed with distilled witch hazel (*Hamamelis virginiana*).

*David Hoffmann is a registered herbalist and FNIMH in the USA, who is the author of *Medical Herbalism.*

5. Herbal Formulas for Acne, orally use by Dr. S. Chen*

Oregon grape, *Mahonia aquifolia*	15%
Sarsaparilla root, *Smilax species*	10%
Burdock root, Arctium lappa	10%
Nettle seed, *Urtica dioica*	10%
Yellow dock root, *Rumex crispus* 10%	
Bupleurum root, *Bupleurum falcatum, Bupleurum chinesis*	10%
Mashmallow root, *Althaea officinalis*	10%
Chaste tree, *Vitex agnus-castus*	10%
Saw palmetto, *Serenoa repens*	10%
Licorice, *Glycyrrhiza glabra*	5%

Dose: 2-3 capsules, three times a day before meals.
*The author of this book

Case Study: Above multi-herb formula for acne

A 26-year-old young man, moderate papulopustular acne on his face, forehead, upper back and upper chest that had not had satisfactory results from erythromycin treatment. He also had constipation. He took dairy, ham, beef, chicken and pork regularly, and favored BBQ once a month. He was a PhD candidate in a stressful academic life. He didn't take any vitamins, minerals or supplements. Blood tests revealed that he had no abnormalities. Stool fecal fat analysis indicated elevated fecal fat levels.

The Anti-Acne Protocol for this patient:

A. Generally do:

1. Diet: Avoid or eliminate all kinds of acne trigger foods, such as dairy, lamb, beef, chicken and simple carbohydrates. Avoid chocolate, cocoa, caffeine, cheese, and butter. No fried and BBQ food. No fatty and trans-fatty foods. Eat more organic and high fiber vegetables & fruits, more soybean products such as tofu, tofu cake, soybean peel, etc.
2. No smoking.
3. To avoid exogenous hormones, use only organic animal products.
4. Avoid iodized salt and swimming in chlorinated water.
5. Cleanse the skin gently on a daily basis with Calendula herb soap.
6. Keep doing exercise and get fresh air regularly.
7. To combat stress, take a break every 10-15 minutes for every 2 hours on computer work.
8. It is necessary to have 7-8 hour of sleep per night.
9. It is healthy to have one bowel movement per day.
10. Drink 8 cups of water per day, more during exercise.
11. As soon as you feel a pimple coming on, wrap an ice cube in saran wrap and hold it on the new pimple for a few minutes.

B. Orally use:

B-complex 50, 1-2 cap a day with meals, for stress and skin.
Vitamin A, 10,000 IU, 1 pill two times a day with meals, for acne.
Vitamin E, 400 IU, 1 softgel a day with meals, for acne.
Magnesium, 200 mg, 1 cap a day, before bedtime, for stress and constipation.
Flax seed oil, high lignan, 1000 mg, 3 softgels/day, for acne and constipation.
Aloe vera, 4 oz/day orally, one hour before bedtime, for constipation and acne.
Pearl barley powder, two tablespoons a day, for acne.
Acidophilus, 10 billion, 1 capsule, two times a day, for acne.
Above herbal formula, 3 capsules, three times a day, for acne.

C. Topically use:

Apply 15% tea tree oil to each skin lesion on the face, upper back and upper chest, two times a day.

After a month on the above protocol, this patient saw a 70% reduction in the number of acne lesions, all papulo-pustular lesions disappeared, with only red papules on his face and upper chest remaining. His constipation went away and his stress improved. Three months later, this patient indicated that no skin lesions were left on his upper chest and upper back, and only two small red papules remained on his forehead. In a follow-up call two years later, he said that when he eats well, experiences less stress, is sleeping well, and has regular bowel movements, he has no more pimples—only the scarring markers remain.

PART 2

AYURVEDA HERBAL MEDICINE for ACNE

Ayurveda, this term is taken from the Sanskirt words *ayus*, meaning life or life span, and *veda*, meaning knowledge. It is a holistic approach to health that is designed to help people live long, healthy, and as well-balanced lives. It has been practiced in India for thousands years and has recently become popularly in Western cultures. The basic principle of Ayurveda is to prevent and treat disease by maintaining balance in the body, mind, and consciousness through proper thinking, diet, and lifestyle, as well as herbal formulas.

Ayurvedic herbs for acne are as following,

Ayurvedic name: **Aloe vera** (This herb is also used in India commonly)
Scientific name: *Aloe vera linn*
English name: Aloe vera
Topical action: It takes care of marks left behind by pimples that have dried away. It restores the former sheen of the skin.

Ayurvedic name: **Arjuna**
Scientific name: *Terminalia arjuna*
English name: Arjun
Topical action: It has excellent effects on facial skin problems such as acne and freckles.

Ayurvedic name: **Badaam**
Scientific name: *Amygdalus communis*
English name: Almond
Topical action: Its oil that is a good laxative. It also replenishes the skin that lost nutrients.

Ayurvedic name: **Bergamot**
Scientific name: *Citrus bergamia*
English name: Bergamot
Topical action: It has been used since centuries to cure sores, skin rashes and acne.

Ayurvedic name: **Chandana**
Scientific name: *Santalum album*
English name: Sandalwood
Topical action: It has cooling properties. Its mild fragrance brings freshness to the affected part. It purifies the blood and prevents further outbreaks of acne.

Ayurvedic name: **Guggulu**
Scientific name: *Commiphora wightii, Commiphora mukul*
English name: Guggul
Topical action: It reduces triglycerides and cholesterol (LDL) level which helps in decreasing the oil secretion on the skin. It improves acne.

Ayurvedic name: **Gulab**
Scientific name: *Rosa centifolia*
English name: Rose
Topical action: It's extract which known as *gulab jal* is extensively used in Ayurvedic medicine for cooling the body. It helps in reducing the Implammation of the pimples.

Ayurvedic name: **Haldi**
Scientific name: *Curcuma longa*
English name: Turmeric
Topical action: It has many known benefits since several millennia. It is very useful for all skin ailments, including psoriasis. But *haldi* must be avoided by people who suffer from gallstones, jaundice and liver diseases.

Ayurvedic name: **Jamun** or **Jambul**
Scientific name: *Syzgium cumini*

English name: Indian blackberry or black plum
Topical action: It has typical purple acid, which neutralizes the alkaline content
of the pus in the pimples.

Ayurvedic name: **Kapoor**
Scientific name: *Cinnamonum camphorum*
English name: Camphor
Topical action: It is a cooling agent and provides numbness to the painful areas
of pimples.

Ayurvedic name: **Lodhra**
Scientific name: *Symplocos crataegoides*
English name: None
Topical action: It reduces side-effects of acne, such as skin rashes. It also helps
in good movement of bowls.

Ayurvedic name: **Papaya**
Scientific name: *Carica papaya*
English name: Papaya
Topical action: It has excellent properties for reducing pimples by direct
application on them. Moreover the papain contained in
papaya that helps in digestion and purifies the blood.

Ayurvedic name: **Pudina**
Scientific name: *Mentha arvesis*
English name: Mint
Topical action: Its leaves have good cooling properties, and are used as anti-
inflammatory agent.

Ayurvedic name: **Rai** or **Sarson**
Scientific name: *Brassica hirta*
English name: Mustard (white)
Topical action: It is a known herbal laxative. It relieves the digestive system and
thus helps in acne cure.

Ayurvedic name: **Santra**
Scientific name: *Citrus aurentium*
English name: Orange
Topical action: Its peel contains essential oils that can kill the bacterial cells
forming the pus. It has anti-inflammatory properties.

Ayurvedic name: **Vacha**
Schientific name: *Acorus calamus*
English name: Calamus
Topical action: Clamus oil is volatile. It relieves the pain of pimples and it also has antibacterial properties to prevent further contagion.

Topical treatment in Ayurveda for acne

1). Applying jamun (*Syzgium cumini*) seeds rubbed with water on the pimples will reduce the growth of the pimples.

2). Taking powders of roasted mustard seeds, orange peels and chiraunji (*Buchanania latifolia*) in equal proportions. To grind them into a very fine constitution. This mixture is applied to the face.

3). To squash a properly ripened and soft papaya in water. Massage the whole face with this paste. The paste will begin drying up after about fifteen to twenty minutes. At this juncture, wash the face with clean water and wipe it with a rough towel. Then apply either sesame or coconut oil on the face.
Continuation of this procedure for a week will help a lot in removing the pimples and their residual marks from the face. Apart from that, the face will look moister and get a youthful sheen.

4). Rubbing the face with the peel of an orange also shows good results.

5). To make a paste of jayphal (nutmeg) and red chandan (red sandalwood).
Apply this on the face to reduce pimples.

6). Preparing a mixture of neembu (lemon), black kasondi (coffee pods or java beans) and eatracts of the tulsi (basil) and dry it in the sun. It will become more viscous when it is dried. Apply it on the face in this concentrated form. This acne formula is helpful in acne cure.

7). One more method of combating pimples is to wash the face with buttermilk at least twice a day.

8). A very simple formula is to put the roots of the neem (*Azadirachtha indica*) in water and apply this concoction on pimples. This method also gives fast relief from pimples.

9). To make a paste of 10 grams of besan (flour of chicpea) and 10 grams of haldi (turmeric) in dahi (curds). Applying this paste on the face using massage techniques. Let the paste dry on the face, and then wash it with plain water. This method provides relief within seven days of continuous application.

10). A paste of lodhra (*Symplocos crataegoides*),dhania (coriander) and vach (*Acorus calamus*) also promises results within seven days. This is one of the best acne treatment.

11). To extract the milk of the sharp thorns of the semal tree (cotton tree, *Bombax ceiba*). Applying this milk on the pimples directly and wash after it is dried off. Continue this process for just three days to get results.

12). Add a spoonful of salt in a bowl with hot water. Apply this with a rough towel On the face as through you are sponging the face. Remember to keep your eyes closed during this application. After each application, wring off the excess water from the towel. This is a mildly painful process as the salt will create a tingling sensation with the open areas of the pimples. However, you will obtain sure results in ten days.

13). To make a paste of masoor dal (red lentils) with milk, camphor and ghee. Apply this mixture on the face. This will not only reduce the pimples, but also take care of the pockmarks that can remain when the pimples are dried off. This is the best acne treatment.

14). Another method that can be employed if you have to socialize is to apply a paste of fine powder of dried orange peel in rose water. This will not only remove the pimples quickly but also improve the texture of the skin.

15). To make a paste of lemon juice, milk and kalaunji (seeds of fennel flower) in very fine powder form. Apply this paste on the face at night when retiring to bed. In the morning, wash the face with lukewarm water. This method is a quick way to eradicate pimples and can be used if you have to go to a party or a function.

16). Mix a cup of milk with a cup of lemon juice. This mixture requires a time of ageing. Hence prepare it in the early morning and apply it when going to bed at night. Wash the face the next morning and wipe it with a rough towel. Continue this application for a couple of days until you see signs of relief. This acne formula is helpful in acne cure.

PART 3

TRADITIONAL CHINESE MEDICINE (TCM) for ACNE

Applying the treatment via Traditional Chinese Medicine based on differential diagnosis in case of acne.

A. Clinical Types of Acne

1. Lung Meridian Wind-Heat Type

Signs and Symptoms

> red papules with pruritus and pain, or with pustules on the forehead, nose, temporal, cheeks and chin regions.
> Patients feel thirsty and crave more water. They may also be constipated, and their urine may exhibit dark yellow color.

Features of Tongue and Pulse

> Patient's tongue appears red with a thin, yellowish coating.
> Pulse: taut and slippery.

Principles of Treatment

> Dispelling wind and clear the lungs

Formula

Principally, **Pipa Qing Fei Yin** (Loquat and lung clearing formula).
Add or reduce herbs depending on specific signs and symptoms.

Sheng Di, Dried Rehmannia root, *Radix rehmanniae*		*30.0g*
Dan Pi, Moutan bark, *Cortex moutan radicis*		*12.0g*
Chi Shao, Red peony root, *Radix paeoniae rubra*		*12.0g*
Zhi Mu, Anemarrhena rhizome, *Rhizoma anemarrhenae*		*10.0g*
Sang Bai Pi, Mulberry bark, *Cortex mori radicis*		*12.0g*
Pi Pa Ye, Loquat leaf, *Folium eriobotryae*		*9.0g*
Huang Qin, Scutellaria root, *Radixs Scutellariae*		*12.0g*
Sheng Shi Gao, Gypsum, *Gypsum fibrosum*		*30.0g*
Sheng Gan Cao, Licorice root, *Radix glycyrrhizae*		*6.0g*

Preparation, Dosage and Administration:

Two options

a. Boil raw herbs in distilled water for oral use. Formulation shown provides one-day's use to be administered in two equal doses, half in the morning and half in the evening. It takes about one hour to cook, and make herbal decoction.
b. For easier use, dissolve concentrated herbal granules in hot water to be drunk as a tea in two equal doses, as described above.

2. Damp-Heat in Gastrointestinal Tract Type

Signs and Symptoms

Greasy skin affecting the face, scalp, upper chest and upper back areas. The lesions show redness, swelling and pain. Or lesions may appear as pustules. In addition, there may be bad breath, constipation and dark yellow color of urine.

Features of Tongue and Pulse

The tongue appears red with a coating of yellow and greasy fur. Pulse: slippery and rapid.

Principles of Treatment

> Clearing away heat, eliminating dampness and detoxification of blood.

Formula

> Principally, **Yin Chen Hao Tang**. Add or reduce herbs depending on specific signs and symptoms.

Yin Chen, Capillaris, *Artemisiae capillaris herbae*	*10.0g*
Zhi Zi, Gardeniae, *Gardeniae fructus*	*10.0g*
Sheng Di, Dried Rehmannia root, Radix rehmanniae	*15.0g*
Che Qian Zi, Plantago, *Plantaginis semen*	*12.0g*
Ze Xie, Alisma, *Alismatis rhizome*	*10.0g*
Da Huang, Rhubarb, *Radix et Rhizoma rhei*	*6.0g*
Sheng Yi Yi Ren, Coix, *Coicis semen*	*30.0g*
Bai Hua She She Cao, Spreading hedyotis herb, *Herba hedyotidis diffusae*	*30.0g*
Sheng Shan Zha, Hawthorne, Crataegus *pinnatifida*	*15.0g*
Gan Cao, Licorice, *Glycyrrhizae radix*	*6.0g*

Preparation, Dosage and Administration:

Two options

a. Boil raw herbs in distilled water for oral use. Formulation shown provides one-day's use to be administered in two equal doses, half in the morning and half in the evening. It takes about one hour to cook, and make herbal decoction.
b. For easier use, dissolve concentrated herbal granules in hot water to be drunk as a tea in two equal doses, as described above.

3. Phlegm Stagnation and Blood Stasis Type

Signs and Symptoms

> Dark red lesions on the face, upper back and central part of upper chest, accompanied by papules, abscesses, cysts and various sized scars. Also, draining sinuses which occur for prolonged and are difficult to cure. Patient may complain of poor appetite and bloating.

Features of Tongue and Pulse

> The tongue appears dark red with a coating of yellow and greasy fur. Pulse: taut and slippery.

Principles of Treatment

> Dissolving dampness, resolving phlegm, activating circulation, and eliminating stagnation.

Formula

> Principally, **Er Chen Tang mixed with Tao Hong Si Wu Tang**.
> Add or reduce the herbs depending on specific signs and symptoms.

Gui Wei, Chinese angelica, *Radix angelicae sinensis*	*12.0g*
Chi Shao, Red peony root, *Radix paeoniae rubra*	*12.0g*
Tao Ren, Peach kernel, *Semen persicae*	*10.0g*
Hong Hua, Safflower, *Flos carthami*	*10.0g*
Chao San Leng, Stir-fried Common burreed tuber, *Rhizoma sparganii*	*12.0g*
Chao E Zhu, Parched Zedoary Root, *Rhizoma curcumae*	*12.0g*
Kun Bu, Kelp, *Thallus laminatiae seu Thallus ecklonia*	*15.0g*
Hai Zao, Seaweed, *Sargassum*	*15.0g*
Xia Ku Cao, Common Selfheal fruit-spike, *Spica prunellae*	*15.0g*
Chen Pi, Tangerine Peel, *Pericarpium citri reticulatae*	*12.0g*
Zhi Ban Xia, Prepared pinella tuber, *Rhizoma pinellae*	*12.0g*

Preparation, Dosage and Administration:

Two options

a. Boil raw herbs in distilled water for oral use. Formulation shown provides one-day's use to be administrated in two equal doses, half in the morning and half in the evening. It takes one hour to cook, and make herbal decoction.
b. For easier use, dissolve concentrated herbal granules in hot water to be drunk as a tea in two equal doses, as described above.

4. Disharmony of Chong and Conception Meridians Type

This type of acne caused by a hormonal imbalance, which affects female menstrual cycle. Patient has irregular menstruation and dysmenorrheal.

Signs and Symptoms

skin lesions are apparently link to menstruation cycle Inflammatory papules occur or worsen prior to period of menstruation, accompanied by moodiness, distending pain in the breast, constipation and irregular menses.

Features of Tongue and Pulse

The tongue appears red with a coating of yellowish and greasy fur Pulse: taut and thready.

Principles of Treatment

Soothing the liver by nourishing *yin*, and regulating the *Chong* and *Ren* meridians.

Formula

Zi Yin Shu Gan Tang, and its modification.

Chai Hu, Chinese Thorowax root, *Radix bupleuri chinese*		*12.0g*
Yu Jin, Aromatic turmeric root, *Radix curcumae*		*15.0g*
Bai Shao, White peony root, *Radix paeoniae alba*		*12.0g*
Nu Zhen Zi, Glossy privet fruit, *Fructus ligustri lucidi*		*15.0g*
Han Lian Cao, Yetbadetajo herb, *Herba ecliptae*		*30.0g*
Yi Mu Cao, Motherwort herb, *Herba leonuri*		*12.0g*
Fu Lin, Indian Bread, *Poriae*		*15.0g*
Shan Zha, Hawthorne berry, *Fructus crataegi*		*12.0g*
Ze Xie, Oriental Waterplantain rhizoma, *Rhizoma alismatis*		*12.0g*
Gan Cao, Licorice, *Radix Glycyrrhizae*		*6.0g*

Preparation, Dosage and Administration:

Two options

    a. Boil raw herbs in distilled water for oral use. Formulation shown provides one-day's use to be administrated in two equal doses, half in the morning and half in the evening. It takes one hour to cook, and make herbal decoction.

    b. For easier use, dissolve concentrated herbal granules in hot water to be drunk it as a tea in two equal doses, as described above.

B. Herbal Modifications for Varies Manifestations of Acne

In addition to one of above recommended formulas, add certain herbs for oral use to treat the following specific signs and symptoms.

1. Acne with **thirsty (polydipsia)**
   Add Sheng Shi Gao, Gypsum, *Gypsum fibrosum*
   Tian Hua Fen, Trichosanthes, Radix trichosanthis

2. Acne with **constipation**
   Add Da Huang, Rhubarb, *Radix et Rhizoma rhei*

3. Acne with rashes and **more pustules**
   To add Zi Hua Di Ding, Viola, *Herba violae*
   Bai Hua She She Cao, Spreading heyotis herb,
   Herba Hedyotidis diffusea,
   Jin Yin Hua, Honeysuckle flower, *Flos ionicerae*
   Ye Ju Hua, Indian Dendranthema flower, *Flos chrysanthemi indici*

4. For female patient whose acne **worsens before or during menstrual period**
   Add Xiang Fu, Nutgrass galingale rhizoma, *Rhizoma cyperi*
   Yi Mu Cao, Motherwort herb, *Herba leonuri*
   Dang Gui, Chinese Angelica, *Radix Angelicae sinensis*

5. The female acne patient with **dysmenorrheal**
   Add Yi Mu Cao, Motherwort herb, *Herba leonuri*
   Ze Lan, Shiny bugleweed herb, *Herba lycopi*

6. Acne with **cysts and pus/abscess**
   To add Bei Mu, Fritillary bulb, *Bulbus fritillariae*
   Chuan Shan Jia, Pangolin scale, *Squama manitis*
   Zao Ci, Chinese Honeylicust Spine, *Spina gleditsidae*
   Ye Ju Hua, Wild chrysanthemum flower, *Flos chrysanthemi indici*

7. Acne with **nodules or cysts that are difficult to heal**
   Add San leng, Burreed tuber, *Rhizoma sparganii*
   E Zhu, Aeruginous turmeric rhizome, *Rhizoma curcumae*
   Zao Ci, Chinese Honeylocust spine, *Spina gleditsiae*
   Xia Ku Cao, Common selfheal fruit-spike, *Spica prunellae*

8. Acne with **bloated and his/her tongue appears thick coating**
   Add Shan Zha, Hawthorn Fruit, *Fructus crataegi cuneatae*
   Ji Nei Jin, Chicken's gizzard skin (stir-fried),
   Endothelium corneum gigeriae galli
   Zhi Shi, Immature bitter orange, *Fructus aurantii immaturus*

9. Acne with **pruritus**
   Add Bai Ji Li, Puncturevine Caltrop Fruit, *Fructus Tribuli*
   Jiang Can, Stiff silkworm, *Bombyx Batryticatus*
   Chan Tui, Cicada slough, *Periostracum Cicadae*

10. Acne with **oily skin**
    Add Bai Zhu, Largehead atractylodes rhizome,
    Rhizoma atractylodis macrocephalae
    Shan Zha, Hawthorn fruit, *Fructus crataegi cuneatae*

C. Patent Chinese Herbal Formulae for Acne

Following **are** patent herbal formulas that have been successfully used by herbalists in China for hundreds to thousands of years

1. *Qing Huo Yi Fei Wan Formula*

   Herbs:

   Huang qin, Baical skullcap root, *Radix scutellariae*
   Zhi Zi, Cape jasmine fruit, *Fructus gardenia*
   Qian Hu,Hogfennel root, *Radix peucedani*
   Ku Shen, Lightyellow sophora root, *Radix sophorae flavescentis*

Tian Hua Fen, Snakegourd root, *Radix trichosanthis*
Jie Geng, Platycodon root, *Radix platycodi*
Zhi Mu, Common anemarrhena rhizome, *Rhizoma anemarrhenae*

Good for cooling fire, clearing lung meridian, and cleansing soreness.
To treat wind and heat in lung meridian type of acne.
Dosage and administration: Orally, 6.0 g, 2-3 times a day.

2. *Lian Qiao Bai Du Wan Formula*

    Herbs:

    Jin Yin Hua, Honeysuckle flower, *Flos lonicerae*
    Zhi Zi, Cape jasmine fruit, *Fructus gardenia*
    Huang Qin, Baical skullcap root, *Radix scutellariae*
    Bai Xian Pi, Densefruit pittany root-bark, *Cortex dictamni*
    Lian Qiao, Weeping forsythia capsule, *Fructus forsythia*
    Chi Shao, Red peony root, *Radix paeoniae rubra*
    Chan Tui, Cicada slough, *Periostracum cicadae*
    Fang Feng, Divaricate saposhnikovia root, *Radix saposhnikoviae*
    Da Huang, Rhubarb, *Radix et rhizoma rhei*

    Good for purging heat, detoxifying blood and clearing pathogenic fire.
    To treat wind and heat in lung meridian type of acne.
    Dosage and administration: Orally, in accordance with label directions.

3. *Xiao Bai Du Gao Formula*

    Herbs:

    Pu Gong Ying, Dandelion, *Herba taraxaci*
    Da Huang, Rhubarb, *Radix et rhizoma rhei*
    Huang Bai, Amur cork-tree, *Cortex phellodendri*
    Chi Shao, Red peony root, *Radix paeoniae rubra*
    Jin Yin Hua, Honeysuckle flower, *Flos lonicerae*
    Ru Xiang, Frankincense, *Olibanum(* Stir-baking with vinegar)
    Mu Bie Zi, Cochinchina momordica seed, *Semen momordocae*(Smashed)
    Chen Pi, Dried tangerine peel, *Pericarpium citri reticulatae*
    Tian Hua Fen, Snakegourd root, *Radix trichosanthis*

Bai Zhi, Dahurian angelica root, *Radix angelicae dahuricae*
Dang Gui, Chinese angelica, *Radix angelicae sinensis*
Gan Cao, Licorice root, *Radix glycyrrhizae*

Good for purging heat, removing toxins, subduing swelling and cleansing soreness. To be used to treat wind and heat in lung meridian type of acne.
Dosage and administration: Orally, 10-20g, two times a day

4. *Dang Gui Ku Shen Wan* Formula

Herbs:

Dang Gui, Chinese angelica, *Radix angelicae sinensis*
Kushen, Lightyellow sophora root, *Radix sophorae flavescenis*

Good for purging heat, dispelling dampness and removing toxins. To be used to treat acne of dampness and heat in stomach meridian and intestine meridian type.
Dosage and administration: Orally, taken in accordance with label directions

5. *Fang Feng Tong Sheng Wan* Formula

Herbs:

Fang Feng, Divaricate saposhnikovia root, *Radix saposhnikoviae*
Jing Jie, Fineleaf schizonepeta, *Herba schizonepetae*
Ma Huang, Ephedra, *Herba ephedrae*
Bo He, Peppermint, *Herba menthae*
Shan Zhi Zi(Zhi Zi),Cape jasmine Fruit, *Fructus gardeniae*
Lian Qiao, Weeping forsythia capsule, *Fructus forsythia*
Dang Gui, Chinese angelica, *Radix angelicae sinesis*
Chuang Xiong, Szechwan lovage rhizome, *Rhizoma chuangxiong*
Bai Shao, White peony root, *Radix paeoniae alba*
Bai Zhu, Largehead atractylodes rhizome, *Rhizoma atractylodis macracephalae*
Jiu Da Huang, Rhubarb(stir-fried with wine), *Radix et Rhizoma rhei*
Mang Xiao, Mirabilite, *Natrii sulfas*
Sheng Shi Gao, Gypsum, *Gypsum fibrosum*
Huang Qin, Baical skullcap root, *Radix scutellariae*

59

Jie Geng, Platycodon root, *Radix platycodi*
Hua Shi, Talc, *Talcum*
Gao Cao, Licorice root, *Radix glycyrrhizae*

Good for dispelling wind, purging heat and removing toxins. To be used to treat acne of dampness and heat in stomach meridian and intestine meridian type.
Dosage and administration: Orally, 6.0-9.0 g, 1 to 2times a day

6. *Da Huang Zhe Chong Wan* Formula

    Herbs:

    Shu Da Huang, Rhubarb(stir-fried), Radix et Rhizome rhei
    Tao Ren, Peach seed, *Semen persicae*
    Huang Qin, Baical skullcap root, *Radix scutellariae*
    Bai Shao, White peony root, *Radix paeoniae alba*
    Sheng Di Huang, Rehmannia root, *Radix rehmanniae*
    Ku Xing Ren, Bitter apricot seed, *Semen armeniacae amarum*
    Tu Bie Chong, stir-fried Ground beetle, *Eupolyphaga seu steleophaga*
    Shui Zhi, Leech(stoving), *Hirudo*
    Mang Chong, Gadfly(dried and stir-fried), *Tabanus*
    Gan Qi, Dried lacquer, *Resina toxicodendri*
    Qi Cao, Northest black chafer(shad dried, stir-fried with sweet rice, *Larva holotrichiae*
    Gan Cao, Licorice root, *Radix glycyrrhizae*

    This formula works particularly well to enhance blood circulation, resolve blood stasis and resolve masses. To be used to treat severe acne of phlegm stagnation and blood stasis type.
    Dosage: Orally, four pills, 3 times a day.

7. *Dan Shen Tong Jiao Nang* Formula

    Herb:

    Dan shen, Tanshinone, *Saliva miltiorrhiza* extract

    Good for purging heat, as an anti-infective, detoxifying blood, enhancing blood circulation, and resolving blood stasis. To be used to treat all types of acne. Dosage and administration: Orally, taken in accordance with label directions.

8. *Mei Hua Dian She Dan* Formul
   It is good for purging heat, removing toxins, resolving blood stasis and resolving masses. To be used to treat all types of acne.
   Dosage: Orally, two pills, 3 times a day.

D. Acupuncture and Massage for Acne

1. Acupuncture Therapy

   Main Points: Quchi (LI 11), Hegu(LI4), Zusanli(ST36), Neiting(ST44), Sibai (ST2), Dicang(ST4), Jiache(ST6).
   Side Points: Feishu(BL13), Xinshu(BL15), Weishu(BL21), Dachangshu(BL25).

   The above points are stimulated bilaterally, with the needles to remain in points on the face and the four limbs for 30 minutes. Needle transmission should be carried out once every 10 minutes. Use purgation style needles for 3-5 minutes, which will provide acupuncture sensation from Shu points on the patient's back.
   Then withdraw the needles. Needle one time every other day for a 10-treatment course of therapy.

2. Ear Acupuncture Therapy

   Points: Lung, Nei Fen Mi, Jiao Gan, Brain, Cheek, Forehead.

   Add Spleen point in cases of acne with seborrhea, large intestine point in cases with constipation, and uterus and liver points in cases with irregular menses. Choose four to five of the above points for each treatment and rotate insertion points. Or use the technique of leaving small beans covered by tape at each point in lieu of inserting needles. Then press the beans with a finger at each point for 3 to 5 minutes, 2 to 3 times a day. Beans should be changed once every 2-3 days over a 5-time course of treatment.

3. Massage Therapy

   For promoting flow of Chi and blood, and for balancing the viscera via massage of meridians, usually once a week.

(1). For adolescent patients with acne a. Use the thumb to press along the medial-posterior knee down to beneath the medial ankle, which is the Foot Shao Yang Kidney Meridian, repeat 10 times. b.Use the thumb to press along the posterior knee, via the lateral ankle, and on to the small toe, which is the Foot Tai Yang Bladder Meridian. Repeat 5 times. c.Stimulate the points Quchi (LI 11), Hegu (LI 14), Lieque (LU 7), and Feishu (BL 13) with the thumb or finger, which is acupressure.

(2). For acne with imbalanced of stomach and intestine function Using the palm or thumb, press/rub along beneath the anterior knee (lateral aspect of tibia bone), via anterior ankle, down to the top side of foot, and stop at lateral aspect of the second toe, which is the Foot Yang Ming Stomach Meridian. Repeat 10 times. **Important**: remember to massage from knee to foot/toe, **not** in reverse order. Also, press the point Zusanli (ST36) with the thumb for 30 seconds to create the sensation of soreness, numbness, distention, and heaviness being spread to the deep area of this point.

E. Topical Treatment for Acne

1. *Dian Dao San* Herbal Lotion

   Formula:

Da Huang, Rhubarb, Radix et Rhizoma rhei	7.5g
Sulphur	7.5g
Limewater	100.0ml

   The above two herbs must be finely powdered and be mixed well with limewater.

   Use: Apply to acne skin lesions, and then wash off area with warm water. Use 30-60 minutes, one to two times a day. Patient should take oral anti-acne herbal medicine at same time.

2. *Si Huang Xi Ji* Herbal Lotion

   Formula:

Da Huang, Rhubarb, *Rhizoma Rhei*	*50.0g*
Huang Qin, Baicai scutellaria root, *Radix scutellariae*	*50.0g*

Huang Bai, Amur cork-tree, *Cortex phellodendri*	*50.0g*
Liu Huang, Sulphur	*15.0g*
Distilled Water	*500 ml*

The sulfur must first be dissolved in 75% alcohol and then placed into distilled water, mixed with the above three herbs, and stir well.

Use: Apply to acne skin lesions, 4 to 6 times a day. Patient should take oral anti-acne herbal medicine at the same time.

3. *Cuo Kang Gao* Herbal Cream

Formula:

Huang Qin, Baical Skullcup Root, *Radix Scutellariae*
Huang Bai, Amur Cork-tree, *Cortex Phellodendri*
Huang Lian, Golden Thread, *Rhizoma Coptidis*
Bing Pian, Borneol, Dryobalanops aromatic Gaertn. f.
Other ingredients: stearic acid, glycerin monostearate, stearyl alcohol, glycerin, minerals oil, laurocapram, retinoids, menthol, and vitamin B6.

When used in conjunction with oral anti-acne herbal medicine, it is highly effective against acne papules that are accompanied by increased redness, swelling and pustules.

Use: Apply topically to acne skin lesions and then wash face with warm water.

4. *Jin Huang Gao* herbal Ointment (20%)

Formula:

Da Huang, Rhubarb, Radix et Rhizoma rhei	*75.0g*
Huang Bo, Amur Cork-tree, Cortex phellodendrii	*75.0g*
Jiang Huang, Turmeric, Rhizoma curcumae longae	*75.0g*
Bai Zhi, Dahurian angelica root, *Radix angelicae dahuricae*	*75.0g*
Tian Nan Xing, Jackin-thepulpit tuber, *Rhizoma arisaematis*	*30.0g*
Chen Pi, Dried tangerine peel, *Pericarpium citri reticulatae*	*30.0g*
Cang Zhu, Atractylodes rhizome, *Rhizoma atractylodis*	*30.0g*
Hou Pu, Officinal magnolia bark, *Cortex magnolia officinalis*	*30.0g*
Tian Huan Feng, Snakegourd root, *Radix trichosanthis*	*150.0g*

Gan Cao, Licorice root, *Radix glycyrrhizae*   30.0g
Fan Shi Lin, Vaseline   500.0g

Grind the above 10 herbs into a fine powder and mixed well. Place100g of the mixed powdered herbs in 500g of Vaseline.

Use: Apply topically, twice a day. Especially useful for cases of s, acne with nodules, cysts, and abscesses. Patients still need to take oral anti-acne herbal medicine at same time.

5.   *Liu Shen Wan* Formula

Formula:

Niu Huang, Cow Bezoar, *Calculus Bovis*
Zhen Zhu Fen, Pearl powder, *Pernulo*
She Xiang, Musk, *Moschus moschiferus L.*
Chan Su, Toad Venom, *Venerum Bufonis*
Bing Pian, Borneol, *Dryobalanops aromatic Gaertn. f.*
Xiong Huang, Rabiagar, *Realgar*

This is a well-known formula that has been using in China for more than 270 years. It was formulated by the family of the Chinese herbalist, Dr.Lei, in the dynasty Qing, and has been used orally or topically to cured many thousands patients who suffered from sore throat, strep throat, canker sore, laryngitis, tonsillitis, hoarseness, furuncle, carbuncle, folliculitis, ulcer of tongue and other ailments.

Use: Grind pills into powder and mixed well with distilled water or vinegar into a poultice for topically use, twice a day. Patient should take oral anti acne herbal medicine at same time.

6.   *Fresh Herbal Lotion*

Formula:

Ma Chi Xian, Pursiane herb, *Herba portulacae* or Xian Ren Zhang, Cactus, *Opuntia stricta* or Lu Hui, Aloe, *Aloe vera L. var chinesis (Haw) Berger*

Choose either the above as a multi-herb formula or use any single herb. Mash into a poultice.

Use: Apply topically to acne skin lesions topically for 20 minutes, twice a day. For best results, patient should take oral anti-acne herbal medicine at the same price.

7. *Dodder Seeds Herbal Lotion*

Formula:

Tu Si Zi, Dodder seed, *Semen cuscutae*	*30.0g*
Distilled Water	*500ml*

Place the dodder seeds in distilled water and cook for about 40 minutes that will yield 300 ml of an herbal lotion.

Use: Wash the acne rashes with this lotion, or wet 4-5 layers of gauze and cover the acne rashes with this lotion for 10-15 minutes of each treatment, twice a day, over a 7-day course. Then stop the treatment for 3 days. Finally, restart the process for an additional 7 days wash until there is significant improvement or complete healing. For best results, It is necessary that the patient take oral anti-acne herbal medicine at the same time.

8. *Green mung bean & Chrysanthemum Lotion*

Formula:

Lu Dou, Green mung bean	*30.0g*
Ju Hua, Chrysanthemum flower, *Flos chrysanthemi*	*10.0g*
Bai Fu Zi, Giant Typhonium Rhizoma, *Rhizoma typhonii gigantei*	*10.0g*
Bai Zhi, Dahuricae Angelica Root, *Radix angelicae dahuricae*	*10.0g*
Bing Pian, *Dryobalanops aromaticae gaertn. f.*	*5.0g*
Distilled water	*1000ml*

Cook above green mung bean and three herbs for 30 minutes. Finally, add the Bing Pian into this lotion for additional 10 minutes. Bing Pian does not need to be cooked and it dissolves quickly in the hot herbal lotion if it is in a granule form.

Use: Drain out the lotion and wash the acne rashes with gauze for 10 minutes at a time, two times a day. Discard remaining herbs.

9. *Aloe Vera lotion or Gel*

This supplies multi-enzymes and vitamin A and E to the epidemic cells, which helps to nourish the damaged cells and speed healing. It is good for mild type of acne vulgaris. The patient should take an oral anti-acne herbal formula at the same time.

10. *Huang Bai Fu Qian Mask* (for severe acne only)

Formula:

Huang Qin, Baical Skullcap Root, *Radix Scutellariae*	*20.0g*
Bai Zhi, Dahurian Angelica Root, *Radix Angelicae Dahuriae*	*20.0g*
Bai Fu Zi, Prepared Common White Monkshood	
Daughter Root, *Radix Aconiti Lateralis Preparata*	*20.0g*
Qian Shi, Gordon Euryale Seed, *Semen Euyales*	*20.0g*

The above four herbs must be dried and finely powdered, then made into a paste with cold water.

Use: In cases of acne with pus. The pus should be cleared up first before applying this mixed-herb paste, Apply herb paste to the entire face, leaving it in place for 20 minutes, then wash off. Do it once a week. In addition to applying the above herb paste, the patient should also take the following herbal formula orally.

Formula for oral use

Ye Ju Hua, Wild Chrysanthemum Flower,	
Flos Chrysanthemum Indici	*10.0g*
Lian Qiao, Weeping Forsythia Capsule, *Fructus Forsythiae*	*10.0g*
Huang Qin, Baical Skullcap Root, *Radix Scutellariae*	*10.0g*
Bai Hua She She Cao, Spreading Hedyotis Herb,	
Herba Hedyotidis Diffusae	*10.0g*
Ce Bai Ye, Chinese Arborvitae Twig and Leave,	
Cacumen Platycladi	*10.0g*
Xuan Shen, Figwort Root, *Radix Scrophulariae*	*10.0g*
Zao Jiao Ci, Chinese Honeylocust Spine, *Spina Gleditsiae*	*10.0g*
Yi Yi Ren, Coix Seed, *Semen Coicis*	*30.0g*
Sheng Di Huang, Raw Rehmannia Root, *Radix Rehmanniae*	*30.0g*
Gan Cao, Liquorice Root, *Radix Glycyrrhizae*	*5.0g*

Preparation and use: Cook the above raw herbs with distilled water, making the herb decoction for oral use. This makes into two equal servings, to be taken half in the morning and half in the evening. Use in a 6-week course.

If the acne contains pus, add the following herbs.
Pu Gong Ying, Dandelion, *Herba Taraxaci*
Bai Zhi, Dahurian Angelica Root, *Radix Angelicea Dahuricae.*

If the acne contains hard nodules, add the following herbs.
Zhe Bei Mu, Thunberg Fritillary Bulb, *Bulbus Frtillariae Cirrhosae*
Chuan Shan Jia, Pangolin Scale, *Squama Manitis*

If the acne contains cysts, add the following herbs
Cang Zhu, Atractylodes Rhizome, *Rhizoma Atractylodis*
Xia Ku Cao,Common Selfheal Fruit Spike, *Spica Prunellae*

11. *Rhubarb Mask*

Formula:

Da Huang, Rhubarb, *Radix et Rhizoma Rhei*	*150.0g*
Starch Powder (Medicinal Starch)	*30.0g*

Grind the rhubarb into a fine powder, then mix in warm water with the starch powder to make into a paste.

Use: Apply the paste to the affected area of the face for 30 minutes, then wash off. Use once per day for 10 days. The patient should take oral anti-acne herbal medicine at the same time.

12. *Three flowers Mask*

Formula:

Jin Ying Hua, Honeysuckle Flower, *Flos Lonicerae*	*10.0g*
Ye Ju Hua, Wild Chrysanthemum Flower,	
Flos Crysanthemi Indici	*10.0g*
Mei Gui Hua, Rose Flower, *Flos Rosae Rugosae*	*10.0g*
Zao Jiao Ci, Chinese Honeylocust Spine, *Spina Gleditsiae*	*10.0g*
Bai Fu Ling, Indian Bread, *Poria*	*10.0g*

Dan Pi, Tree Peony Bark, *Cortex Moutan*	*10.0g*
Ce Bai Ye,Chinese Arborvitae Twig and Leaf,	
Cacumen Platyciadi	*15.0g*
Zhen Zhu Fen, Pearl Powder	*5.0g*

Grind above herbs into a fine powder. To make the paste, mix 30g of the resulting powder with warm distilled water.

Use: Cleanse the facial skin with negative ionic water spray for 20 minutes. Apply the paste all over the face including areas of papulo-pustules or open and closed comedones for 30 minutes, twice a week, in a 6-week course. The patient should take oral anti-acne herbal medicine at the same time.

13. *Qi Guorong Herbal Mask*

Formula:

Da Huang, Rhubarb, Radix et Rhizoma Rhei	60.0g
Liu Huang, Sulfur, Sulphur	40.0g
Huang Bai, Amur Cork-tree, Cortex Phellodedri	40.0g
Zi Cao, Arnebia Root, Radix Arnebiae	20.0g
Bai Zhi, Dahurian Angelica Root, Radix Angelicae Dahuricae	40.0g
Shui Zhi, Leech, Hirudo	20.0g
Tian Nan Xing,Jackin-thepulpit Tube, Rhizoma Arisaematis	20.0g

Grind the dried leech and herbs into a fine powder and mix well, stored in a clean glass bottle.

Use: Combine 5g of the powder mix with one piece of egg white each time to create the mask to cover the face, once a week, over a 4-week course. The patient should take oral anti-acne herbal medicine at the same time.

14. Dr. *Xu Shuhuai's Herbal Mask*

Formula:

Bai Zhi, Dahurian Angelica Root, *Radix Angelicae Dahuricae*	*80.0g*
Dan Shen, Danshen Root, *Radix Salviae Mil Tiorrhizae*	*100.0g*
Liu Huang, Sulfur, *Sulfur*	*50.0g*

Da Huang, Rhubarb, *Radix et Rhizoma Rhei*   *50.0g*
Ku Shen, Light yellow Sophora Root,
Radix Sophorae Flavescentis   *50.0g*
Lian Qiao, Weeping Forsythia Capsule, *Fructus Forsythiae*   *20.0g*
Chuan Xin Lian, Common Androgarphis Herb,
Herba Angrographitis   *20.0g*
Pu Gong Ying, Dandelion, *Herba Taraxasi*   *20.0g*
Tian Kui Zi, Muskroot-like Semiaquilegia root,
Radix Semiaquilegiae   *20.0g*

Grind the above dried herbs into a fine powder, mix well, and store in a clean glass bottle.

Use: It is effective for treating acne lesions. And, it should be used with oral anti-acne herbal medicine at the same time.

15. *Cuo Chuang Herbal Tincture*

Formula:

Huang Lian, Golden Thread, *Rhizoma Coptidis*   *15.0g*
Huang Bai, Amur Cork-tree, *Cortex Phellodendri*   *15.5g*
Huang Qin, Baical Skullcap Root, *Radix Scutellariae*   *10.0g*
Di Fu Zi, Belvedere Fruit, *Fructus Kochiae*   *15.0g*
Ku Shen, Lightyellow Sophora Root,
     Radix Sophora Flavescentis   *15.0g*
Chen Pi, Dried Tangerine Peel, *Pericarpium Citri Reticulatae*   *15.0g*
Dan Shen, Danshen Root, *Radix Salviae Mil Tiorrhizae*   *20.0g*
Bing Pian, Borneol, *Dryobalanops aromatic Gaertn. f.*   *10.0g*
Jia Xiao Zuo, Metronidazole   *2.0g*
Luo Nei Zhi, Spironolactone   *1.0g*
Vitamin B6,   *2.0g*

Grind the fist seven herbs into the fine powder and soak in 40-60% alcohol for 7 days. Then filter and add the powdered Borneol, metronidazole, spironolactone and vitamin B6, shake well. Discard remaining herbs.

Use: Applying to the papulo-pustules, open and closed comedones, and pustule lesions. It is particularly effective in cases of adolescent acne. Patient should take oral anti-acne herbal medicine at the same time.

16. *Anti-Seborrhea Herbal Lotion for Washing*

Formula:

Shan Dou Gen, Vietnamese Sophora Root,	
Radix Sophotae Tonkinensis	*15.0g*
Sang Bai Pi, White Mulberry Root-bark, *Cortex Mori*	*15.0g*
Shi Chang Pu, Grassleaf Sweetflag Rhizome,	
Rhizoma Acori Talarinowii	*15.0g*
Wu Bei zi, Chinese Gall, *Galla Chinensis*	*15.0g*
To Gu Cao, Intricate Clematis Herb,	
Herbra Clematidis Intricatae	*15.0g*
Zao Jiao Ci, Chinese Honeylocust Spine, *Spina Gleditsiae*	*15.0g*

Cook the above herbs with distilled water 400 to 500ml about 30 minutes and drain the resulting herbal lotion into a container. Discard remaining herbs. Add 1000ml of warm water to the lotion and wash the face with it once per day, to reduce the facial oil. Patient should take oral anti-acne herbal medicine at the same time.

17. Anti-Facial Oil Herbal Lotion for Washing

Formula:

Zao Jiao, Chinese Honeylocust, *Fruit Fructus Gleditsiae*	*30.0g*
To Gu Cao, Intricate Clematis herb,	
Herbra Clematidis Intricatae	*30.0g*

The Chinese Honeylocust should be ground before cooking. Then cook the two herbs with distilled water 2000 ml about 30 minutes and drain the herbal lotion to a container. Discard remaining herbs.

Use: Wash face, once a day.

18. *Herbal Steaming Therapy*

It is effective for all types of acne, especially for severe cases which show pimples on the upper chest or upper back.

Formula:

> Ku Shen, Lightyellow sophora root, *Radix sophorae flavescentis*
> Bai Jiang Cao, Whiteflower Patrinia Herb, *Patrinia villosa Juss.*
> Bo He, Mint, *Mehtha canadaensis L.*
> Bai Hua Shen She Cao, Spreading Hedyotis Herb, *Oldenlandia diffusa (willd.) Roxb*
> Pu Gong Ying, Dandelion, *Taraxacum mongolicum hand.-Mazz*
> Ye Ju Hua, Chrysanthemum flower, *Flos chrysanthemi indici*
> Zi Hua Di Ding, Viola Yedoensis, *Viola philipica Cav.*
> Yin Chen, Capillary Wormwood Herb, *Artemisia capillaris Thunb.*
> Xian He Cao, Hairyvein agrimony, *Agrimoniae pilosae Ledeb.*
> Hu Zhang, Giant Knotweed Rhizome, *Rhizoma polygonum cuspidati*

Cook the herbs for 40 minutes, and then steam areas of pimples for 30 minutes, once a day. If cases of acne with pus/cysts, cleanse pus and contents of the cysts surgically after the steaming. Use for a 7-day course, then withhold treatment for two days before resuming use for another.

F. Food Therapy for Acne

Both foods and herbs are from key components of Traditional Chinese Medicine (TCM). Acne patients should eat more fresh vegetables and fruits every day. Organic foods are the best choice.

Suitable Foods

Vegetables: Celery, spinach, cucumber, cabbage, baichai, asparagus, radish, winter melon, tomato, broccoli, carrots, cauliflower, lettuce, eggplant, kales, beets, sprouts, bell peppers, bitter melon, peas, soybeans

Fruits: Apple, pear, grapes, grapefruit, coconut, honeydew melon, loquat, strawberry, blueberry, black cherry, mulberry, orange, banana, water melon, water chestnut and lemon

Meats and fish: Lean meat of pork, duck, goose, donkey, quail, snake, hedgehog, pigeon, rabbit, river snail, river crab, ocean crab, clams, abalone, edible frog, lobster, octopus, mullet, cuttlefish, yellow fish, scallop, loach, sea eel, mackerel, bass, reeves shad, butterfish, silver fish, salmon, shark, soft shelled turtle, carp, cruciate carp and sea cucumber

Other foods: Mushrooms, to fu, bean curd, seaweed, konbu

Eat more brown rice, millets, corn, buckwheat, barley, oats, and whole grain bread.

Suitable Beverages:

1. Chrysanthemum, *Flos chrysanthemi* flower tea. Place dried chrysanthemum flower 3.0 g in 6-8 oz of hot water for 3-5 minutes. Drink, refill it one to two times a day. Good for clearing away pathogenic heat and for improving visual acuity.

2. Xia Ku Cao, Selfheal Herb, *Prunella vulgaris L.* tea. Useful for clearing away pathogenic heat, improving visual acuity, dispersing stagnation, and reducing swelling. Dosage: 9-15 g decocted in water for a single daily oral dose.

3. Gui ling Gao. Contains primarily Gui Ban (*Carapax et plastrum testudinis*), Tu Fu Ling (*Rhizoma smilacis glabrae*), and honey. Available in herbal gel form in a can, ready to drink. Also available in tea-bag form; dosage: 1-2 bags at a times, 3 times daily. Either form is good for depleting dampness, clearing away heat and detoxifying blood.

4. Mung bean beverage. Place 25-30 g of dried mung bean in 1.2 liters of water and cook for 60 minutes to create a beverage. Stevia or other sweeteners may be added to enhance taste. This daily dose is useful for clearing away heat and detoxifying blood.

The above four beverages are popularly used in China by patients with acne and should be combined with other herbal medicines for oral and topical use.

Important points to remember:

According to the Traditional Chinese Medicine, the pathological cause of acne in most acne cases is pathogenic heat that triggers excessive secretion of the sebaceous glands, thus blockage of pilo-sebaceus duct and promoting bacterial infection. Usually, incorrect diet, stress, sleepless, constipation, temperamental, genetic, humid and hot climate may rise body pathogenic heat. This chain of events forms the basis for the selections of foods to be consumed or avoided by the patients, as described below.

Foods to Avoid

Meats: *lamb, sausages, ham, any fried, roasted or barbequed meats.*
Beverages: *alcohol* and coffee

Tonics: most herbal energy boosters, such as red and panax ginseng, deer antler, cordyceps, astragalus, ephedra, yohimbe, guarana, maca, catuaba, avena sativa, horney goat weed, and whey protein.

Others: chocolate, trans fats, fatty foods, dairy foods, eggs, sweets, ice cream, French fries, baked or fried chips and crackers, all kinds of roasted seeds, all kinds of roasted nuts, greasy foods, spicy foods, hot peppers, white or black peppers, mustard, curry, cinnamon bark, raw garlic, raw onion, raw green onion, ginger, durian (a fruit from Southeast Asia). The foods and a fruit underlined above, when consumed, increase body heat markedly and are thus considered to be "hot foods"* according to Traditional Chinese Medicine (TCM). They should be avoided by patients with *heat types* of acne.

*Hot foods: it means that foods play a hot role when they enter the body.

Foods to eat in Reduced Quantities

The following foods, when consumed, increase the body heat gently and are considered to be "warm food"* according to Traditional Chinese Medicine (TCM). They should be eaten in reduced quantities by patients with excessive heat type acne, damp and heat type acne.

Meats and fish: beef, chicken, turkey, dog, cat, deer, camel, sparrow, shrimp, eel, trout, catfish, cat fish, chub, blow fish, rudd, hairtail, cuttle, silver carp, grass carp, abalone, turtle, sea horse, blood clam, and sea cucumber.

Vegetables: cooked white radish, young baichai, leek, cauliflower, cooked lotus root, pickled potherb mustard, coriander, baby fennel, toon head, pumpkin, basil, shoot, sweet potatoes, konjac, sweet jing cai, sword bean, allium macrostemon bunge, elsholtzia and crown daisy.

Fruits: mango, lemon, guava, Kumquat, thoreau fruit, bergamot, waxberry, rambudan, bilberry fruit, sakyamuni, wampee, papaya, pamogranate, dates, apricot, lychee, plum, longan, hawthorn berry, cherry, coconut meat, dark plum, plum, honey peach, tico berry, seabuckthorn berry, wild pepper and trifoliate orange.

Grains: sweet rice, black rice, purple rice, sago, wheat germ, oats, and sorghum.

Non-roasted nuts: pistachios, chestnuts, walnuts, pine nuts, date palm, betel nuts, and Korean pine seeds.

*Warm foods: it means that foods play a warm role when they enter the body.

Beneficial Foods for Certain Types of Acne

All kinds of lightly and highly "cool/cold foods"* and "neutral foods"* which include most vegetables, peas, beans, certain soy foods and fruits, which foods rich in vitamins A, B, C, D, E, fiber and zinc are beneficial for acne patients with lung meridian wind-heat type acne and in gastrointestinal damp-heat type acne. Such as **buckwheat** and **pearl barley** are good for damp and heat type acne; **young dishcloth gourd, lotus root, bitter melon** and **water melon** are helpful for all heat types of acne.

*cold/cool foods:
It means that foods play a cool/cold role when they enter the body.

*Neutral foods:
It means that foods play neither cool/cold nor warm/hot roles when they enter the body.

Patients with phlegm station and blood stasis type acne should avoid greasy foods, avoid eat too fast and over eating, less salted, acid foods and cold fruits to eat, and no smoking, which are the key pathogenic triggers for these types of acne. Food such as **tangerine peels** and **water chestnut** are particularly beneficial in nourishing spleen chi, depleting dampness, softening hard masses, and eliminating phlegm and dampness associated with these types of acne.

The foods are beneficial for phlegm and dampness:
Pearl barley, corn, millet, rice, Gorgen fruit, red bean, broad bean, mooli, cowpea, seaweed, black mushroom (Shitaike), jellyfish, quail, kidney bean, cabbage, yamaimo, winter melon kernel, apricot, lychee, chestnut,lemon, cherry, red bayberry, bergamot, pepper, garlic, green onion, onion, ginger, chub, trout, hairtail, loach, finless eel, river shrimp, lamb, beef, dog, and chicken. Above foods are good for phlegm dampness and blood stasis type acne.

The foods are beneficial for blood stasis:
Lotus, onion, mushroom, Hericium erinaceus (Hou Tou Gu, a mushroom), tree mushroom, seaweed, kudzu root, konjac, needle mushroom, Rhizome of old world arrowhead (Zi Gu), rape, black bean, pineapple, orange, phyllanthus emblica (Yu Gan Zi), hawthorn berry, water chestnut, roxburgh rose, and pork heart. Above foods are good for dampness and blood stasis type acne also. A few ounces of red wine to drink and doing exercise everyday are advised.

For acne patients with disharmony of Chon and Conception meridians, **rose flower**, a flower to relax the liver and nourish the kidneys, improve mood, relieve the early stage of depression, reduce tenderness in the breast area, is highly recommended. Dosage: 4 to 6 buds mixed with green tea in each cupful.

For acne patients with disharmony of Chong and Conception meridians, **mulberry**, a sweet fruit to nourish Yin and blood, to make more fluid and sooth the intestines.

For acne patients with disharmony of Chong and Conception meridians, **goji berry**, a sweet fruit to nourish the liver and kidneys and to strength Yin and Yang, especially Yin.

For acne patients with disharmony of Chong and Conception meridians, **wheat**, a grain to nourish the heart and kidneys, to invigorate the spleen, and regulate the blood.

For acne patients with disharmony of Chong and Conception meridiants with sallow complextion, hot flashes, and mood swings, **dates**, a sweet fruit to reinforce the spleen and stomach, to replenish Chi and blood, to tranquilize the mind, adjust Yin Chi and Wei Chi, and to harmonize the properties of herbal medicines.

PART 4

INTRODUCTION ON
THREE TRADITIONAL MEDICINES

A. An Introduction to Western Herbalism

Herbalism is a traditional medical practice based on the use of plants and plant extracts. The scope of herbal medicine is extended to include fungal and bee products, as well as minerals, shells and certain animal parts. Pharmacognosy is the study of medicines derived from natural sources.

People on all continents have used hundreds to thousands of indigenous plants for treatment of ailments since prehistoric times. Medical herbs were found in the personal effects of *Otzi the iceman*, whose body was frozen in the Otztal Alps for more than 5300 years. These herbs appear to have been used to treat the parasites found in his intestines.

The ancient Greeks and Romans made medicinal use of plants. Greek and Roman medical practices, as preserved in the writings of Hippocrates and—especially—Galen, provided the pattern for later western medicine. Hippocrates advocated the use of a few simple herbal drugs—along with fresh air, rest, and proper diet. Galen, on the other hand, recommended large doses of drug mixtures—including plant, animal, and mineral ingredients. The Greek physician complied the first European treatise on the properties and uses of medicinal plants, *De Materia Medica*. In the first centuries AD, Dioscorides wrote a compendium of more than 500 plants that remained an authoritative reference into the 17th century. Similarly important for herbalists and botanists of later centuries was the Greek book that founded the science of botany. Theophrastus' *Historia Plantarum*, written in the fourth century BC.

The uses of plants for medicine and other purposes changed little in the early medieval Europe. Many Greek and Roman writings on medicine, as on other subjects, were preserved by hand copying of manuscripts in monasteries. The monasteries thus tended to become local centers of medical knowledge, and their herb gardens provided the raw materials for simple treatment of common diseases. At the same time, folk medicine in the home and village continued uninterrupted, supporting numerous wandering and settled herbalists. Among these were the "wise-women", who prescribed herbal remedies often along with spells and enchantments. It was not until the late Middle Ages that women who were knowledgeable in herb lore became the targets of the witch hysteria. One of the most famous women in the herbal tradition was Hildegard of Bingen. A twelfth century Benedictine nun, she wrote a material text called *Cause and Cures*.

Traditional western medicine evolved mostly from the ancient Greeks, who were strongly influenced by Egyptian and Middle Eastern civilizations. Western herbal medicine also has roots in the indigenous practices of the British Isles and ancient Roman traditions.

The fifteenth, sixteenth, and seventeenth centuries were the great age of herbals, any of them available for the first time in English and other languages rather than Latin or Greek. The first herbal to be published in English was the anonymous *Grete Herball* of 1526. The two best-known herbal works in English were *The Herball or General History of Plants* (1597) by John Gerard and *The English Physician Englarged* (1653) by Nicholas Culpeper.

The second millennium, however, also saw the beginning of a slow erosion of the pre-eminent position held by plants as sources of therapeutic effects. This began with the Black Death, which the then dominant Four Element medical system proved powerless to stop. A century later, Paracelsus introduced the use of active chemical drugs. The rapid development of chemistry and other physical sciences, led increasingly to the dominance of chemotherapy—chemical medicine—as the orthodox system (conventional medicine) of the twentieth century.

In the modern society, herbs of the western herbal medicine tradition are the subject of increasing interest in the medical community. Research is currently being conducted in the use of medical herbs for various medical conditions. Single herbal formulas and multi-herbal formulas are suggested purposed, such as improvement for general support circulatory, respiratory, digestive, urinary, nervous, endocrine and skin systems processes of the human beings, even animal diseases. Herbs are also used to purportedly remove waste and toxins from the body cells or topically to promote healing of the skin, as a complementary and alternative medicine to the conventional medicine.

The researches on single herb in Western herbalism have gained a series of success by the influence and guide of the conventional medicine. Such as, clear up each herb's actions and pharmacology, clinical trials, indications and usage, contraindications, precautions and adverse reactions, drug interactions and dosage, described accurately by the evidences from the scientific studies. This is an excellent model in the herbal community. But, the research on the clinical effectiveness of multi-herbal formulas, toxicology of herbs, compatibility and interaction between herb to herb, herb to chemical medicine, etc. and make more effective new herbal formulas to enrich the science of formulae (prescriptions) in the herbology, which have yet to be proved by more patients uses, and more trained-well medical practitioners' practices. In brief, Western herbalism, a treasure of all human beings, needs to develop rapidly with conventional medicine.

B. An Introduction to Ayurvedic Medicine

Ayurvedic medicine (also called Ayurveda) originated in India and has evolved there over thousands of years. Ayurvedic medicine is an extraordinary traditional medicine over the world. It integrates and balances the body, mind, and spirit, which prevent disease and promote wellness. Ayurvedic medicine treats certain diseases in multiple systems of the body, and effectively for physical and mental health problems also. A chief aim of Ayurvedic practices is to cleanse the body of substances that may cause diseases, thus reestablish harmony and balance of the body.

Two ancient books, written in Sanskrit more than 2000 years ago, are considered the main texts on Ayurvedic medicine—*Caraka Samhita* and *Sushruta Samhita*. The texts described eight branches of Ayurvedic medicines:

Internal medicine
Surgery
Treatment of head and neck disease
Gynecology, obstetrics, and pediatrics
Toxicology
Psychiatry
Care of the elderly and rejuvenation
Sexual vitality

Ayurvedic medicine is based on the principles that the universe is made up of five elements: air, fire, water, earth and ether. These elements are represented in humans by three *"doshas"*, or energies: *Vata, Pitta,* and *Kapha.*

Vata pertains to air and ether elements. This energy is generally seen as the force, which directs nerve impulses, circulation, respiration, and elimination.

Kapha pertains to water and earth elements. It is responsible for growth and protection. The mucosal lining of the stomach, and the cerebral-spinal fluid that protects the brain and spinal column are examples of *kapha.*

Pitta pertains to fire and water elements that governs metabolism, e.g., the transformation of foods into nutrients. It is responsible for metabolism in the organ and tissue system.

When any of *doshas* accumulate in the body beyond the desirable limit, the body loses its balance. Every individual has a distinct balance, and our health and well-being depend on getting a right balance of the three *doshas("tridoshas"),* which control the activities of the body.

Ayurvedic medicine believes the body's constitution (*prakriti*), which refers to a person's general health, the likelihood of becoming out of balance, and the ability to resist and recover from disease or other health problems. The *prakriti* is a person's unique combination of physical and psychological characteristics and the way of the body functions to maintain health.

Ayurvedic treatment goals include eliminating impurities, reducing symptoms, increasing resistance to disease, and reducing worry and increasing harmony in the patient's life. A process called *panchakarma* that cleanse the body by dispelling *ama, which* is a disease, caused by an undigested food sticks to tissues, interferes with normal functioning of the body. Panchakarma focuses on removinging *ama* through the digestive tract and respiratory system. Enemas, massage, medical oils administered in a nasal spray, and other methods may be used.

Ayurvedic treatments rely heavily on herbs and other plants—including oil and common spices. Currently, more than 600 multi-herbal formulas and 250 single—herbal formulas are included in the Ayurvedic pharmacy.

C. An Introduction to Traditional Chinese Medicine (TCM)

Before the existence of the conventional medicine, human beings depended solely on the herbal medicines and other therapeutic methods to treat illness, pre-illness and preserve health. Such a practice gave rise to the establishment of various kinds of traditional medicine with unique theory and practice, such as Ayurvedic medicine, Arabian medicine, Western alternative medicine, and the Traditional Chinese Medicine (TCM), etc. Among these traditional systems of medicine, Western herbalism, Ayurvedic medicine and the TCM are three extraordinary ones.

With a history of more than 3000 years, the TCM has formed a distinctive system to diagnosis, cure illness and pre-illness. Since the written language in China has been founded, including inscriptions on the bones and tortoise shells of Yin Dynasty (2100-1600 B.C.), records of such diseases in internal medicine as headache and cardiac pain are found.

The first Chinese herbal book, the *Shennong Bencao Jing*, complied during the West Han Dynasty (100 BC), listed 365 medicinal plants and their uses that including mahuang (Ephedra), the shrub that introduced the drug ephedrine to modern medicine.

The Yellow Emperor's Internal Classic was the earliest medical classic extant in China, which appeared in Warring States Period (475-221 B.C.). This book dealt mainly with pathogenic factors, pathogenesis, diagnosis and treatment of disease in internal medicine, summarizing basic theories and clinical practice of the TCM at that time.

Treatise on Febrile and Miscellaneous Disease, a classic medical work in China, written by the outstanding physician Zhan Zhongjing in the East Han Dynasty (3rd century A.D.). This book laid a solid foundation of internal medicine, perfected the pattern of theories, methods, prescriptions and meteria medica, and founded principles of diagnosis and treatment based on overall analysis of symptoms and signs, the cause, nature and location of the illness and patient's physical condition according to the basic theories of the TCM, making great contribution to the development of internal medicine.

Compendium of Materia Medica, a well-known book on Chinese herbal medicine, written by physician Li Shizhen, published in China in 1590. There are 1,892 herbs and 11,096 herbal formulas are described in this book. It is a monumental work in the history of herbal medicine in China.

The TCM approach is fundamentally different from that of conventional medicine. In the TCM, the comprehension of the human body is based on the holistic understanding of the universe as described in Daoism, and the treatment of illness is based on primarily on the diagnosis and differentiation of syndromes (symptom-complexes). Such as acne, a common skin disease, named by conventional medicine. In the TCM, it has mostly four different types (syndromes) which are **lung meridian wind-heat type acne, damp-heat in GI tract type acne, phlegm stagnation and blood stasis type acne and disharmony of Chong and Conception meridians type acne.** Those terms in diagnosis feature a combined of the TCM and conventional medicine. The earliest herbal formula for acne in written language was found an ancient grave in Changsha, Mawangdui, Hunan province of China in 1973. This grave was in the West Han Dynasty, 100 BC.

The basic theories of the TCM describe the physiology and pathology of the human body, disease etiology, diagnosis, and differentiation of syndromes, which includes the theories of yin-yang, five elements, zang-fu organs, meridians-collaterals, Chi (qi), blood, body-fluid, methods of diagnosis, and differentiation of syndromes.

The TCM theories possess two outstanding features, their holistic point of view, and their application of treatment according to the differentiation of syndromes. According to these traditional viewpoints, the zang-fu organs are the core of the human body as an organic entity in which tissues and sense organ are connected through a network of meridians and collaterals (blood vessels). This concept is applied extensively to physiology, pathology, diagnosis, and treatment.

The functional physiological activities of the zang-fu organs are dissimilar, but they work in coordination. There exists an organic connection between the organs and their related tissues. Pathologically, a dysfunction of the zang-fu organs may be reflected on the body surface through the meridians and their collaterals (i.e. blood flowing in the blood vessels near body surface). At the same time, diseases of body surface tissues may also affect their related zang or fu organs. Affected zang or fu organs may also influence each other through internal connections. The TCM treatment consists of regulating the functions of the zang-fu organs in order to correct pathological changes.

Not only is the human body an organic whole, but it is also a unified entity within nature, so changes in the natural environment may directly or indirectly affect it. For example, changes of the four seasons, and the alternations of day and night may change the functional condition of the human body, while various geographical environment can influence differences in body constitution, and so on. These factors must be considered when diagnosis and treatment are given. The principles of treatment are expected to accord with the different seasons and environments.

Application of treatment according to the differentiation of syndrome is another characteristic of the TCM. "Differentiation of syndromes" means to analyze the disease condition in order to know its essentials, to identify the causative facts, the location and nature, and to obtain conclusions about the confrontation between pathogenic and anti-pathogenic factors. In the TCM, differentiation performed to outline the specific principles and methods of treatment because similar diseases may have different clinical manifestations, while different diseases may share the same syndromes. **Treatment in the TCM stresses the differences of syndromes, but not the differences of diseases**. Therefore different treatments for the same disease exist and different diseases can be treated by the similar medical analogy.

Treatments of the TCM include Chinese herbal medicine, acupuncture and moxibustion, therapeutic massage, diet, osteopathy, and Chi (Qi) gong, etc.

Diseases in internal medicine, surgery, gynecology, dermatology, psychiatry, venereology, pediatrics, genesiology, oncology, toxicology, gereology, ear, nose and throat system, even certain diseases in stomatology and infectious disease, which might be treated by the TCM in China. The TCM plays an important role in taking care of pre-illnesses also. By professionals' reports in China, the heavy epidemic of SARS in China in 2003, the Chinese herbal medicine worked with west medicine there, effectively treated many patients with SARS, and successfully saved patients' lives, which firmly proven the TCM is an indispensable medicine in the medical community.

REFERENCES

Bassett IB, Pannowitz DL, et al. A comparative study of tea-tree oil versus benzoyl-peroxide in the treatment of acne. *Med J Aust* 1990; 153:455-458

Carson CF, Riley TV. Antimicrobial activity of the major components of the essential oil of *Melaleuca alternifolia* (Tea Tree oil). *J Appl Bacterial* 1995; 78:264-269

Carson CF, Riley TV. Toxicity of the essential oil of Melaleuca alternifolia or Tea Tree oil. letter; comment. *J Toxicol Clin Toxicol* 1995; 33:193-194

Cox SD, Gustafson JE, Mann CM, et al. Tea Tree oil causes K+ leakage and inhibits respiration in *Escherichia coli*. *Lett Appl Microbiol* 1998; 26: 355-358

Enshaieh S, Jooya A, Siadat AH, et al. The efficacy of 5% topical tea tree oil gel in mild to moderate acne vulgaris: a randomized, double-blind placebo-controlled study. *Indian J Dermatol Venereol Leprol* 2007; 73(1): 22-25

Koh KJ, Pearce AL, Marshman G, et al. Tea Tree oil reduces histamine-induced skin inflammation. *Br J Dermatol* 2002; 147:1212-1217

Magin PJ, Adam J, Heading GS, et al. Complementary and Alternative Medicine Therapies in Acne, Psoriasis, and Atopic Eczema: Results of a Qualitative Study of Patients' Experiences and Perceptions. *J Alt Comp Med.* 2006; 12(5): 451-455

Shapiro S, Meier A, et al. The antimicrobial activity of essential oils and essential oil components toward oral bacteria. *Oral Microbiol Immunol* 1994; 9: 202-208

Magin PJ et al. Topical and oral CAM in acne: A review of the empirical evidence and a consideration of its context. *Comp Ther Med.* 2006; 14(1): 62-76

Frohne D. *Solanum dulcamara L.*(Bittersweet Nightshade)—Der BittersuBe Nachtschatten. Portrai einer Arzneipflanze. *Z Phoytother* 1992; 14:337-342

Ivanovska N, Philipov S. Study on the anti-inflammatory action of berries vulgaris root axtract, alkaloid fractions, and pure alkaloids. *Int J Immunopharmac* 1996; 18:553-561

Bernstein S, Donsky H, Gulliver W, et al. Treatment of mild-to-moderate psoriasis with Relieva, a mahonia aquifolium extract—a double blind, placebo-controlled study. *Am Med Ther* 2006; 13:121-126

Van Loon IM, The golden root: Clinical applications of scutellaria baicalensis Georgi flavonoids as modulators of the inflammatory response. *Altern Med Rev* 1997; 2: 472-480

Zhang J, Shen X. Antioxidant activities of baicalin, green tea polyphenols, and alizarin in vitro and in vivo. *J Nutr Environ Med* 1997; 7: 79-89

Park J, Lee J et al. In vivo antibacterial and anti-inflammatory effects of honokiol and magnolol against propionibacterium sp. *Eur J Pharmacol* 2004; 496:189-195

Chi YS, Lim H, Park H, et al. Effects of wogonin, a plant flavone from scutellaria radix, on skin inflammation: In vivo regulation of inflammation-associated gene expression. *Biochem Phamacol* 2003; 66: 1271-1278

Bojar RA, Holland KT. Acne and propionibacterium acnes. *Clin Dermatol* 2004; 22:375-379

Biju SS, Ahuja A, et al. Tea tree oil concentration in follicular casts after topical delivery: Determination by high-performance thin-layer chromatography using a perfused bovine udder model. *J Pharm Sci* 2005; 94: 240-245

Balambal R, Thiruvengadam KV, et al. Ocimum basilicum in acne vulgaris—a controlled Comparison with a standard regime. *J Assoc Physicians India* 1985; 33: 507-508

Takahashi T, Kokubo R, Sakaino M. Antimicrobial activities of eucalyptus leaf extracts and flavonoids from eucalyptus maculate. *Lett Appl Microbiol* 2004; 39: 60-64

Slobodnikova L, Kost'alova D et al. Antimicrobial activity of mahonia aquifolium crud eatract and its major isolate alkaloids. *Phytother Res* 2004; 18: 674-676

Morsy TA, Rahem MA, et al. Eucalyptus globules (camphor oil) against the zoonotic scabies, sarcoptes scabiei. *J Egypt Soc Parasitol* 2003; 33: 47-53

Willuhn G, Phytopharmaka in der Dermatology. In: *ZPT* 1995; 16(6): 325-342

Li WY, Zhang FC. *Dermatology and Venereal Disease*. Beijing: People's Medical Publishing House, 2004

Brantner A, Lucke W. Influence of physical parameters on the germ-reducing effect of microwave irridation on medicinal plants. *Pharm Ind.* 1995;50 (11): 762-765

Biyun C. The clinical observation of treating acne vulgaris with Xiao Cuo Fang. *J Chinese Medicinal Materials* 2004; 27: 308-310

Morton JF. *An Atlas of Medicinal Plants of Middle America*. Charles C Thomas Pub.USA 1981

Teuscher E, Lindequist U, Biogene Gifte—Biologie, Chemie, Pharmakologie, 2. Aufl., Fischer Verlag Stuttgart 1994

Fetrow CW, Avila RA. *The complete guide to herbal medicines*. Bethlehem Pike, PA: Springhouse Corporation, 2000

Yarnell E, Abascal K, Rountree R. *Clinical Botanical Medicine*. 2nd ed., rev. and expanded. New Rochelle, NY: Mary Ann Liebert Inc., 2009: 5-14

Hoffmann D. *Medical Herbalism, The science and practice of herbal medicine*. Rochester,Vermont: Healing Arts Press, 2003: 439,565,566,578,595

Zhu YF, Zhao HR. In vivo determination of activities in inhibiting propionibacterium acne with Chinese herbs. *Pharma and Clin Res.* 2009, 17(3):224-226

Guo S, Zhang AH, Wei YG. Study on the progress in treating acne with Chinese herbs. *Guid J TCM and Parma* 2009; 15(1): 87-89

Dong MJ, Ni Y. Study on pharmacological action and constituents of Fructus forsythia (Lian qiao) *J Shanxi Chinese Med* 2009; 25(4): 56-57

Ro JY, Lee B, Kim JY, et al. Inhibitory mechanism of aloe single component (Alprogen) on mediator release in guinea pig lung mast cells activated with specific antigen-antibody reactions. *J Pharmacol Exp Ther* 2000; 292:114-121

Hutter JA, Salmon M, Stavinoha WB, et al. Anti-inflammatory C-glucosy chromone from aloe barbadensis. *J Nat Prod* 1996; 59:541-543

Chithra R, Sajithlal GB, et al. Influence of aloe vera on collagen characteristics in healing dermal wounds in rats. *Mol Cell Biochem* 1998; 18:71-76

Heggers J, Kucukcelebi A, et al. Beneficial effect of aloe on wound healing in an excisional wound model. *J Alter Complemet* Med 1996; 2: 271-277

Hamman JH. Composition and application of aloe vera leaf gel. *Molecules* 2008; 13(8): 1599-1616

Yamashita T, Matsumoto T, Yahara S et al. Structures of two new steroidal glycosides, Soladulcosides A and B from Solanum dulcamara. *Chem Pharm Bull* 1991;39:1626-1628

Boll PM. Alkaloidal glycosides from Solanum dulcamara. IV. The constitution of beta—and gamma-solamarine. *Acta Chen Scand* 1963;17:2126

Bluementhal M. *The complete German commission E monographs: Therapeutic guild to herbal medicine.* Austin TX: American Botanical Council; 1998: 232

Dather AM. From medical herbalism to phytotherapy in dermatology: back to the future. *Dermatol Ther* 2003;16(2): 106-113

Jin ZC, Dong ZJ, Zhang GY. Study on 118 cases with acne treated by Chinese herbal steaming therapy. *Gan Su J TCM* 2003; 16(2):23-24

Huang M, Tian LM, Wang WQ. Study on acne on the chest and upper back with Chinese herbal steaming therapy. *Hu Bei J TCM* 2006; 28(10): 39

Qi GY. Study on 150 cases with acne treated by Chinese herbal Masque and Xiao Cuo Tang. *Si Chuan J TCM* 2008; 26(12): 106

Chen TY, Wang P. *The experience in treating acne by Dr. Tongyun Chen.* Beijing: People's Military Medical Press, 2010: 114

www.ingramcontent.com/pod-product-compliance
Lightning Source LLC
Chambersburg PA
CBHW031305280526
45784CB00004B/1990